INSPIRATIONAL BLUEPRINTS FOR PERSONAL SUCCESS – FOR WOMEN

By
Dr Nkem Ezeilo

"How we spend our days is, of course,
how we spend our lives"
Annie Dillard

DISCLAIMER AND/OR LEGAL NOTICES

The information in this book represents the views and opinions of the author as of the date of the publication. The author reserves the right to alter or change her opinion as more information becomes available or new research findings give cause for such a change in opinion. Every attempt has been made to present accurate information in this book; however, this book is for informational purposes only. Neither the author nor her affiliates assume any responsibility for errors, omissions or inaccuracies. If advice of health, legal, financial or related nature is required, you are advised to seek the help of qualified professionals. This book is not intended to be a source of financial, health, legal or accounting advice. You should be aware of any laws which govern business transactions in your country and state. Any reference to any person or business, whether living or dead, is purely coincidental.

FAUNTEEWRITES

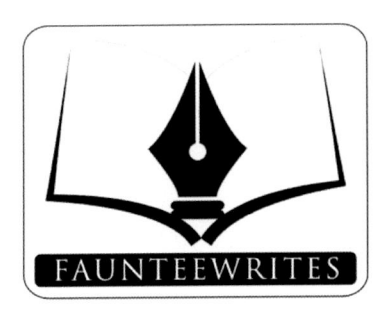

Published by
Faunteewrites Limited
© Dr Nkem Ezeilo 2010 , 2016

Dr Nkem Ezeilo asserts the moral right to be identified as the author of this work.

ISBN : 9780993041761

ALL RIGHTS RESERVED. No part of this book may be reproduced or transmitted in any form whatsoever, electronic or manual including photocopying, recording or by any informational storage or retrieval system without express written, dated and signed permission from the author.

To every woman who knows she could be, do and have more, and desires a roadmap to help her break through every barrier and limitation, to every woman who has a vision of herself as an Empowered, Independent, Resourceful and FREE individual, to every woman who wishes to be a part of 'The New Women's (mental) Liberation Movement ™', this book is for YOU.

Acknowledgements

I wish to express my deepest gratitude to everyone who has helped make this book a reality.

To the great I AM, who daily loads me with blessings, through whom all things are possible.

To David, my son – you give my life so much meaning and inspire me, by your very existence, to continue striving to improve in every way. I love you.

To my parents Gabriel (RIP) and Bernice, and my brothers Ikenna, Chuks and Obinna - you have been such rocks of support especially during the toughest, challenging times of my life. Without you, this book wouldn't exist in the first place. Thank you so much for your continued love and support.

To my sister Doris and my adorable nieces Alexis and Nonye, thank you for bringing smiles to my face each day.

To Faustina Anyanwu of Fauntee Writes Publishing House for your dedication to this project.

To Dion Johnson, the 'midwife' who helped birth this project at this time. Thank you for the paradigm shift you helped me achieve, making this book possible. You're awesome, Coach!

To my coaching clients and readers of my regular newsletters, who continue to support my work with such enthusiasm. I thank you all.

CONTENTS

Day 1: The Power to Choose	01
Day 2: Laying the Foundation	15
Day 3: Success Primers: Habits	35
Day 4: Success Primers: Values	55
Day 5: Success Primers: Responsibility	63
Day 6: Success Primers: Self-Discipline	69
Day 7: Success Primers: Determination	75
Day 8: Use Your Imagination to Succeed	81
Day 9: The Power of your Beliefs	93
Day 10: The Attraction of Gratitude	103
Day 11: Appropriate Action	111
Day 12: The Proper Use of Willpower	119
Day 13: Choose Your Pain And Work With It	127
Day 14: Cure The Worry Habit	135
Day 15: Systems Are the Key to Your Success	143
Day 16: Affirmation	151
Day 17: listening to your inner voice	161

Day 18: Declutter Your Life	169
Day 19: How to Conquer Procrastination	177
Day 20: Do it Now	185
Day 21: How do yous	191
Day 22: Get a mental Workout	199
Day 23: How to be Selfish to Succeed	205
Day 24: Love Thy Neighbour	213
Day 25: How To Overcome indecision	223
Day 26: 3 Steps to Freedom	229
Day 27: How to Make The Most of Your Time	239
Day 28: Why You Should Write Things Down	247
Day29: How to Get Results Through Prayer	255
Day 30: Yes You Can	269
Appendix: How I Overcame Breast Cancer Diagnosis	279
About the Author	285

PREFACE
THE NEW 'WOMEN'S (mental) LIBERATION MOVEMENT' IS HERE or 'Why This Book Was Written'!

This book was written to challenge women everywhere to join 'The New Women's Liberation Movement', and in doing so, to impact and change our world for the better, starting from your world, dear reader.

What IS The New Women's Liberation Movement?

Whatever your impression of the phrase 'Women's Liberation', it's likely to have nothing, or at least very little, to do with The New Women's Liberation Movement.

Hint: this new 'movement' has nothing to do with feminism.

This is a movement which aims to liberate every woman from self-imposed limitations, shackles and obstacles which are preventing her from living life to the fullest. These barriers keep you from achieving success in every area of your life.

They are all within you, so don't be looking outside of yourself for someone or something to be liberated from. The good news is, the solution is all within you as well.

The new 'Women's Liberation Movement' is **a shift in paradigm** that leads to empowerment of the individual woman. A radical shift in mindset to one which enables the woman realise that she is powerful and more than enough in herself to bring about the reality she desires.

The new 'Women's Liberation Movement' aims to help you access this solution so that you can live your best life on a daily basis.

Are you a woman?

Do you feel unfulfilled in certain areas of your life? Does your life lack balance? Do you suffer from a lack of self-confidence or low self-esteem? Would you like to enjoy your relationships, both with your significant other and with your friends, family and colleagues? Do you desire to be financially and emotionally independent? Do you desire total success? Even if you've achieved all the above, do you still feel you could do more, be more, have more?

If you've answered 'yes' to any of these questions, then 'The New Women's Liberation Movement' is for you.

What is this new movement? **It really is a mindset**, a mental program which empowers you to be all you can be, no matter what you do. It is a way of thinking and a way of doing things which is not common... but is guaranteed to bring about results once you wholeheartedly adopt it.

You see, the reason for every challenge and adversity you face can be traced down to yourself directly or indirectly. Of course you have not deliberately put yourself in an undesirable position, but in all likelihood, you have attracted that situation to yourself **by the thoughts** you have allowed to dwell in your mind. Thought determines reality. So if you wish to change the reality you see, you need to go back to the root cause of it: your thoughts.

And no, this is not pollyanna-ish jargon. This is about accepting responsibility for yourself: the moment you accept responsibility for where you are right now, you begin to empower yourself... to make the necessary changes to improve your situation.

When you join in The New Women's Liberation Movement, you will be set to experience Total Success in every area of your life. You will discover the foolproof, tried and tested formula for attracting the things, circumstances and people you desire into your life - and you will be doing this with integrity every step of the way.

How do you join the new Women's Liberation Movement?

By simply deciding to. Decide that - from today - you are turning your life around; you will achieve your goals and dreams; you will enjoy every day you are blessed with; you will be free from your limiting beliefs and negative influences. Once you make this decision in your private, quiet corner (you're not doing this for anyone else, only for yourself), you will become aware of all the resources available around you - to make things happen for you (when the student is ready...)

You must be willing and prepared to do the work involved though.

Laziness (mental, intellectual, emotional and physical laziness) will leave you imprisoned in a world of mediocrity, poverty and misery. Diligence and appropriate ACTION will raise you above your current circumstances and usher you into a world of Total Success and Abundance.

You will know if this message is for you. If it is, if you are indeed ready and feel that enough (mediocrity and just getting by) is enough, then...

Your time is NOW! Get emancipated from your limiting beliefs!

Break through your mental and emotional barriers and begin to experience Total Success!

As a woman thinketh, so is she (mostly because her thoughts determine her actions, which in turn determine her results).

Begin now, your journey, as you work through the following chapters over the next 30 days. Go through it as often as you need to, until these Blueprints become second nature to you.

Your successful future awaits...

INSPIRATIONAL BLUEPRINTS FOR PERSONAL SUCCESS

INTRODUCTION TO THE SECOND EDITION

A lot has happened since I first published this book 6 years ago, making it necessary for me to update it. The bulk of it remains the same, and in fact the events of the past 6 years have proved more than anything the power of the words in this book to change lives, when they are applied.

The most significant events that have happened in the past 6 years include my being diagnosed with breast cancer not once but twice, the second time being told it was at the most advanced and incurable stage (people with the type of diagnosis I was given in 2015 are usually expected to live for a few months afterwards -3 months tops, fewer without chemotherapy).

As I share in the appendix, it's not what they call you that counts or manifests in your life, it's what you answer to.

I chose to answer to LIFE.
I rejected the death sentence handed to me by the medical establishment and told the oncologist that not only was it curable, but I was going to prove it to him.

The principles in this book reveal my strategy for overcoming this most difficult of challenges, and I encourage you to diligently work through the exercises in the book, applying them to your specific condition, for in doing so you too will overcome any challenge before you and will succeed in life.

Success means different things to different women. You get to choose what success means to you. It's your life, after all.

Define success for yourself, and know that in defining it you have just proved that you have what it takes to achieve it.

Knowing this, apply the blueprints in this book and go for it with all you've got!

Your successful future awaits...

INTRODUCTION TO THE FIRST EDITION

I may not have met you before, but there's one thing I know for sure about you: you are a woman who's destined to succeed. You have the potential to be who you want to be, do what you want to do and have the things you want to have in this life. You were born with 'Success' wired into your DNA. Your very genetic fabric has 'Success' woven into it.

THAT, I know to be true about you. Question is, do YOU know this to be true about you?

You deserve to enjoy your life every day. You can enjoy your relationship with your significant other. If you don't have a 'significant other' at this time, you have within you the power to attract just the right person to fill that position – if that's what you desire. You don't have to chase after anyone. You don't have to lose your dignity or self-respect. Just focus on being the very best 'you' possible, and you will attract the right people into your life.

You have the power to attract the job or career you desire, and to prosper in it. You have it in you to be a great leader in every role you're given.

You can enjoy perfect health, abundant energy and zest for life. Every day.

You can be a great mother. You can enjoy enduring and fulfilling relationships with your friends and family.

And you can do all this without feeling guilty about it either! Many times, women feel they must be martyrs, doing their best for others while neglecting themselves.

Well, that's about to change, for you cannot truly give to another until you have given to yourself. You cannot truly love another until you first love yourself.

Plus, it's detrimental to your health to neglect your own needs.

So get it into your head right now that you matter and are worth every minute you spend looking after and nurturing YOU, for that's the ONLY way you can be the best woman, mother, lover, CEO, housewife... whatever role you choose!

What You Can Get Out of This Book

This book will show you how to be free to love yourself. It's one of the most powerful things you could do for yourself and those around you. In doing so, you will discover how to master yourself, how to take control of your life and direct it such that you accomplish your goals, and everyone who crosses your path leaves a better person.

You will learn how to be extremely confident as you discover who you really are, what really counts and what you are capable of. And my goodness are you capable of so so much!

This is not a book to rush through. Read with the intention to begin to rebuild your life in the next 30 days, and when you APPLY the material you learn, you will become unstoppable and nothing will faze you.

How To Use This Book

There are 30 chapters in this book. Devote 15-30 minutes each day for studying this book: read one chapter each day. Study it. Work through it. Do the exercises. Think about what you read. Take notes. Most importantly, ACT on something you've read each day.

What does it take to be totally successful? Success here means real, lasting, fulfilling success, the sort that enriches your life as well as those around you.

It takes **total health in your mind and body.**

In order to succeed, you must be of the correct **mindset** and spiritual **state.** This includes the way you think about and relate to God (the Divine Power living in each of us) It also includes the way you think about and relate to yourself.

Once you get your vital relationships right, every other one falls into place.

Your life right now reflects your predominant mental and spiritual state. This is good news because it means that if you are not happy with the way your life is, **you have the power to change it.**

This book takes you through the blueprints for total success in your personal and professional life. If you wish to discover how to achieve total success in the area of your health, read "**Inspirational Blueprints For Health and Wellness for Women**".

Blueprints are just that – they mean nothing unless you translate them to life by taking appropriate ACTION.

As you go through this book, ask yourself what you can improve in your life from what you've read, and how you can improve it. Write down the ideas that occur to you, and put at least one of them into practice at once. Build up momentum, and you will begin to experience success in small steps. Each baby step of success will encourage you and spur you on to further success.

Discipline will be the bridge between your dreams and their realisation. Make use of it. Discipline will also boost your self esteem to no end so you really want to make use of it.

This book shows you exactly how to cultivate the states which make it conducive for you to take appropriate action, leading to success.

Therein lies the importance of **being in the right state of mind** at all times: your state determines your behaviour (actions). Your behaviour determines your results (success or failure). So your success depends ultimately on what's going on inside you.

Without further ado, let's begin.

PLEASE NOTE
*None of the information you are about to read is worth anything **until you ACT on it**. Therefore, read each word with the full intention of applying what you read. Knowledge is not powerful until you put it into action.*

DAY ONE:
THE POWER TO CHOOSE

"Every choice you make has an end result."
Zig Ziglar

The very first step in changing your life is to choose to do so.

Success is a choice that you make each day, in every area of your life.

Decide to begin making choices whose outcomes you desire.

You can decide the direction your life takes.
You can choose to be a success or not.
Your life today is the way it is because of the choices you have made in the past.

If you feel stuck in an unhappy relationship or job, for instance, it's because you've chosen to remain there. Sounds harsh, but think about it. Why are you stuck? Who's forcing you to remain where you are? There are several options available to you, all it takes is for you to be aware of the fact that there are options available, and then to boldly choose which one to go for.

Doing nothing about your situation is a choice in itself, you know.
Later on in the book you'll discover how to become 'unstuck' in any area of your life, but for now, today, choose and decide to do whatever it takes (that is legal and appropriate), to get out of the rut you're in, and begin to live the full, enjoyable and prosperous life you were created to live. Choose a life of abundance.

You were born free. Choose to use that freedom to live your life to its fullest possible potential.

Sometimes you are not aware of the choices governing the events in your life, but they are there anyway. The aim of this chapter is to open your eyes to the power you have within you to make choices that bring you closer to the quality of life you desire. Hopefully, after reading this, you will be inspired to make good choices every day of your life.

A story to illustrate the point…

I remember the day I decided to become extremely successful. It was my penultimate year in medical school. Up until that time I'd been passing my exams, just sailing along, not putting in much effort and not getting much out as a result. As a matter of fact, I actually failed a couple of exams while I was at it.

The funny thing ('funny weird', that is, not 'funny ha ha') was that without realizing it, **that same mediocre mindset had permeated other aspects of my life.** I felt deeply dissatisfied and wasn't enjoying myself. I was also in the habit of blaming others or external circumstances when things didn't go my way.

Do you know anyone else like this? Anyway, back to the story...

One day I got fed up. This was after failing a second exam. I realised I didn't want to go on living like this. I knew I could do better. It dawned on me that it was my life in question here - nobody could live it for me.

Nobody could achieve the results I desired but me. And right then one of the results I wanted was to excel in my studies. I wanted to be the best medical student that the school had come across. I realised it was up to me to make that happen. Not my parents, not my friends, not even my lecturers.

So on that day I 'took my academic life in my hands' and said in essence, "from this day on I will do what I need to do in order to excel in medical school. I will operate in 'Excel Mode' from now on in every aspect of my life. I'm tired of being mediocre. I will excel. I choose to be extremely successful".

Making a conscious decision to change was enough to get me all fired up. I noticed I now had a hunger to learn more, so I studied my textbooks more. My attitude and actions changed during classes too: I asked more questions, answered more, took more chances to learn things and so on.

That day was the beginning of my experience of '**The Universal Principles of Success**' (see chapter 2). As a result of practising those principles, I passed my finals with distinctions in every subject. I won several awards for being the best student in each subject and then won a special award for being the overall best graduating medical student for the year 1997.

That experience opened my eyes to the power we each have to choose which way our life goes. I hope it opens your eyes, too. You have so much potential in you right now, mostly lying dormant, so much creative power. You can literally become and do anything you want - **you simply need to choose to do so** and then go for it, tolerating no excuses. You have got what it takes to be the best in your field, or the best you can be. There is more than enough room at the top for you when you do choose to excel.

Refuse to be swayed by the opinion of others when making choices for your life because you're the one to live with the consequences of your choices, not them. So stop giving precious energy to wondering what others think about you.

> **Empowering thoughts ...**
>
> One of my clients had major problems with the thoughts she allowed to linger in her mind. They were mostly self-deprecating thoughts. No wonder then that she felt worthless and insecure. She had plenty of dreams and desires but wasn't doing anything about them because she felt she'd fail anyway, and besides, she reckoned, she didn't deserve to have any of them.
>
> As part of the process of change, I asked her to do a series of exercises, which involved 'thought conditioning' or changing her thoughts about herself to positive, empowering ones. It was a form of mental reprogramming.
>
> By the time we finished working together, not only had she become much more confident and positive, she had achieved one of her major goals - she now works abroad in her dream job. It all started when she 'changed her mind', so to speak.

You have the power to choose your thoughts. This is the most important quality you have. Why? Because every single result you see in your life, every effect, every outcome, first started out as a thought.

Your feelings start out as thoughts – notice how your mood depends on your thoughts at any particular time. Your state – the frame of mind which governs your actions at any given time, depends on your current dominant thoughts. Your words start out as thoughts (at least I hope they do!). Your actions thus start out as thoughts too.

Yes, it's true: you ARE what you think.

Your self image, the way you see yourself, is the sum total of the thoughts you hold about yourself, whether they are true or no, whether or not those thoughts have been planted by you or by external influences.

The same is true about the way you see others and the way you see the world around you. It's all about your thoughts.

What you think and the thoughts you allow to dwell in your mind are **all under your control.**

By choosing to allow only empowering thoughts, you choose the way your life turns out. You have free will. You have the power to dream dreams, and the power to choose to make them come true or not.

Stop waiting for someone to come along and make something happen for you. Choose to make things happen in your life!

Right now you have the power to choose thoughts that empower you to be the woman you want to be.

Absolutely nothing and no one stops you from doing so, except yourself.

You have the power to choose how you feel. Isn't that amazing? I think it is. You can't change another person's behaviour, but **you can change your response** to their behaviour. No matter how the other person treats you, no matter what they say to you, no matter what circumstances you find yourself in, the only time any of that stuff affects you is when you let it. Again, you are in the driver's seat here. Your response is your responsibility. It makes sense to choose to respond to things and people in a way that leaves you feeling great on the inside, self-respect and dignity intact.

You can choose how to spend your time. You have goals and dreams, right? Each moment you live, you are either doing something that's taking you towards your dreams or taking you away from them.

When you think of time that way, you'll spend it more wisely. You'll realise that you can't afford to waste any of it. Even your fun and leisure activities will be purposeful.

It all starts with conscious choice on your part.

Time is one of your most precious assets (your health is another one, but that's the topic of another book...), and once it's gone, it's gone. So it is vital that you use your time wisely. Guard it ferociously – if you don't value your time, no-one else will. So don't let others impose themselves on you at a time you've set aside to do something else. Be in control of the time you've got.

Choose to use it well.

You can choose what you eat. Each time you put something into your mouth, you are either nourishing your body and getting healthier or you're destroying it. There's no halfway house here.

Think about that next time you're about to eat anything. **Every seed of action reaps a result.** What sort of results will your current choices yield?

A lot of the health problems facing the world today would be solved if individuals took responsibility for what went into their mouths. There's no escaping it – what you eat either empowers you or it doesn't.

Once you realise this truth, your life will take on a renewed energy. You will know that you alone are in control of your future. You will step up and be the boss of you, your appetite and your eating habits.

You can choose what you say. You can choose how you respond to another person's words. You can choose whether to speak or not. Sometimes it is better not to say anything than to say something and regret it later.

Do you now realise how powerful you are?

Do you now realise that you hold your destiny in your hands? You are either in control of your life, or else someone else is. It depends on who you choose to give control of your life to. The power to choose whose life you're going to live is yours.

Take your life back today. Commit to living a better life from this moment. Take responsibility for your choices and their outcomes. Change the ones that don't work and keep moving on.

It's your choice.

EXERCISE

- GAP (Grab a pen) - write in the space for 'Notes'. Find yourself a quiet space for this. You want to be free from distractions.

- Write a statement describing your life as it is right now.

- Ask yourself "What choices have led to this result?" – ask this about each outcome you have noted in the statement above.

- Write down these thoughts.

- Write down a statement describing your life **as you'd like it to be** - your ideal life. Don't limit yourself here: write what your life would be like if you had no limitations whatsoever.

  Your imagination is where the first creation happens. Always. So start from there to create the sort of person you desire to be.

- What sort of person would you have to be, in order to live that ideal life? What sorts of things would you have to do, say, wear, feel?

- These things you've written above are all external reflections of the thoughts you'd need to have in order to experience your ideal life. So the final question is: what thoughts would you have to have (about yourself, about the world, about others, about any relevant issue) in order to bring about the outward results you desire?

- Choose to make this new way of thinking your default mindset, and don't let anyone steer you off course.

- Come back to this exercise any time you forget or feel discouraged. Remind yourself that by virtue of having the power to choose your thoughts, you have the power to choose your outcomes. So today (and every day henceforth) you will make good choices (in terms of what you think, say and do.)

NOTES

"Man's power of choice enables him to think like an angel or a devil, a king or a slave. Whatever he chooses, mind will create and manifest."
Frederick Bailes

DAY 2: LAYING THE FOUNDATION
10 UNIVERSAL PRINCIPLES OF SUCCESS

"Success doesn't come to you...you go to it."
Marva Collins

This world is an amazing place. We are all connected in one way or another. The principles you are about to discover are the ones I learned back in 1995 while still in medical school. I had never heard of such success 'gurus' as Napoleon Hill, Anthony Robbins, Wallace Wattles, Charles Haanel. Yet I discovered that the topics I wrote about and spoke about were the same things they had written and spoken about, albeit using different language sometimes.

My main 'success manual' which led me to discover the following principles was the Bible. Most of the extraordinarily successful people I have studied since the early 90s has vouched for the power of the words contained in the Bible to change lives,   including all the men mentioned above.

The great thing about the Bible is that you do not have to subscribe to any particular religion for its teachings to work. They are principles, just like gravity, and thus work when you apply them correctly, regardless of your background or religious affiliation. This is because the Bible is not a religious or theological book. It's a serious psychological manual teaching about man and his relationship with his powerful subconscious mind.

So these principles will work for you whether or not you're a christian or other religious affiliation. Since you seek a better life, you have everything to gain by plugging into these principles and applying them diligently to your daily life.

I decided to put these principles into words when I realised they were applicable to areas of life other than just the academic arena. The principles outlined below are the same ones I teach my clients to apply in order to raise the level of their game. Read this chapter and use the same principles to create success in your life today. They work, and this book is all about helping you achieve results.

Success comes as a result of forming certain habits, and maintaining them. Consistency is key. As is discipline. To succeed, you need to be a certain type of person. Don't be discouraged if you are not yet that type of person. With practice, any woman can become a successful person. The successful person thinks in a certain way, talks in a certain way, and acts in a certain way. Therefore these are the areas in which you must apply discipline if you are to experience massive success in your life – thoughts, words, actions.

This chapter outlines 11 of those characteristic ways

that highly successful women behave. Do not be fooled by their simplicity. When done properly, these principles work. They take your life to another level. Don't take my word for it though. Act on them for yourself and see what happens.

Any woman who consistently applies these principles to any area of her life will experience success in that area.

1. **Vision:** Have a clear picture of what exactly it is you want to achieve or become. Keep this picture at the top of your mind at all times. Doing something you want to do, because you want to do it, will motivate you to succeed at it. Start with the end in mind.

   Your imagination is your workshop. This is where you design the life you desire. There are always two creations to everything - the first happens in the workshop of your mind (your imagination), and the second is the physical manifestation of the blueprint you've designed in that workshop.

   Begin today to design the life you desire. If you don't have a clear design and direction for your life, chances are **you're living someone** else's vision, someone else's design. Someone or something else is in control of your life.

   So get to work. Set aside some time **today** to begin creating the life of your design. Set aside a bit of time each day to review your design, add more clarity, adjust any bits that don't quite fit and so on. Have fun with this. You only get one shot at this life. Make it count.

2. **Belief:** Believe without a shadow of a doubt that you can do it. Believe that you will succeed. Believe that God/the Universe - whatever you choose to call the Higher Power that created you and sustains you... is helping you get what you want. Stay away from negative influences (people, books/articles, anything negative), that make you doubt your ability to succeed. Surround yourself with things that remind you that you can, and will, succeed.

If you must doubt anything, **doubt your doubts.** And why not? They hold you back from reaching outside the box to achieve your true potential. They keep you from seeing your true worth. They keep you with the other crabs in the bucket and keep you from rising above the mediocre. So doubt any thought that holds you back or puts you down, and choose to believe and accept only thoughts of good about yourself and your abilities.

Believe you can succeed in that business venture. Believe you can get that promotion. Believe you can attract Mr Right, if that's what you desire. Believe you can write that book. Whatever your mind conceives, whatever you heart desires, BELIEVE it can come to pass.

You see, what you believe becomes your reality. As you work on your design (see 1 above), believe that the design you're working on can actually be your reality. Believe that you deserve to succeed. You should - you were created in God's image and He 'don't make no junk', as someone once said . That powerful image knows only success. That's you.

You were born to succeed. You've got it in you to succeed. You must believe this, and don't let anyone or any circumstances tell you anything different.

No matter what you seek to accomplish, you actions won't have any power unless they're backed up with faith/belief.

Whatever you desire, believe it's possible for you. Armed with this belief, you can now apply the remaining principles in confidence that each step is moving you closer to bringing your dreams to reality.

3. **Responsibility:** You are responsible for your future. You alone are responsible for the outcome of your efforts. Don't look for anyone to blame. Ask for help as you need it, but remember the final decision is up to you. It's your life, after all.

The beauty of accepting responsibility is that it empowers you to make the necessary changes to your life. When you realise that you're responsible for the outcomes you experience, it makes you wiser in the choices you make.

Your life becomes richer in every sense. In your business, you know you are responsible for outsourcing or delegating tasks that would be better done that way. You're responsible for marketing your wares. You're responsible for applying for that job you desire. You're responsible for choosing a self-image that is congruent with the results you desire. You're responsible for making yourself attractive and appealing first on the inside (which means no guilt – seek forgiveness, forgive yourself if necessary, love yourself, then move on; no self-loathing, no man-bashing, love others unconditionally, expecting nothing back from them).

Take responsibility for your future, and when you succeed, then victory will be sweeter.

4. **Affirm:** Make a habit of saying out loud what you hope to achieve. Speak of it in the present tense, e.g., 'I **am** fit and trim', as opposed to 'I will be fit and trim'. If you feel awkward speaking out loud to yourself, write down the affirmation. Then look at it (or better still, rewrite it) several times each day, at least three times a day. This helps your

mind stay focused on the goal. It also builds your self-belief and confidence.

One verse that really helped me propel my results to the stratosphere, is this one: "if you say to this mountain, be removed and be cast in the sea, and you don't doubt, but **believe that what you say comes to pass, you will have what you say"**. Jesus said that. I chose to believe it. Then I started to speak it out loud. I'd say 'the things I say happen'. Then I'd say what I wanted to happen, and I believed (still do) that the things I said (and say) do indeed happen.

I did this whether or not the current physical reality agreed with what I was saying. You see, the law has said that if I speak with faith what I say, will happen. So I started speaking stuff with faith.

Once, when I was still new in business, I entered a rough patch. (I'd stopped affirming stuff - which you'll be tempted to do when things go well) and my bank account was nearly empty. So I decided to start speaking things into being. I started to say 'Thank God for my overflowing bank account and booming business', and things like that. (Note that this affirmation is based on one of Seven Natural Laws, which I discuss in another book – your affirmations must be based on truth otherwise you won't believe them and they won't be effective. Later in this book you'll learn how to make affirmations effective.). I backed my words with faith and took action by going a-prospecting.

In less than 48 hours, 'out of the blue' I had two orders for my highest priced products (at the time they cost over £1000.00 each).

Nobody can tell me this stuff doesn't work!

Watch what you say. Always. Quit saying negative things about yourself or others, your circumstances or theirs. You know that design you came up with at the beginning? Speak it into being. With gratitude. Keep on speaking it into being, and back it all with some action steps (which become clearer to you as you affirm your belief that your design is coming to pass).

This is another ingredient in the recipe for total success. **Your words must line up with your thoughts and actions.**

5. **Commitment:** Make a firm commitment to action. Decide to take whatever steps you need to take to help you achieve your goals. Then honour the commitment you've made. Too often we find it easy to keep our commitments to others while neglecting to keep our commitments to ourselves. This pattern has to change if you're to succeed in life.

Integrity is central to your success, and integrity starts with YOU. Commit to your own success. Decide that failure is not an option (bearing in mind that failure = quitting). When you master integrity with yourself, you'll find it even easier to be a person of integrity with others.

True commitment is much more than just being interested in something happening. It's that spirit of 'no turning back', that attitude of steely determination that helps you overcome all obstacles on your way to your breakthrough. It's that spirit of discipline that makes you do what you have to do even when you don't feel like doing it.

No obstacle can stand in the way of the woman who is truly, fully committed to a given course. Be that woman.

6. **Set a SMART goal:** Now that you know what you want to achieve or become, you need to define it by making it a goal. Your goal has to be

- **S**pecific,
- **M**easurable (you need a standard to help you know when you've achieved it) and **M**otivational (it's got to inspire you and keep you motivated)
- **A**ttainable and **A**ttractive

- **R**ealistic (no point setting an unrealistic goal such as "I want to be a millionaire this evening") and
- **T**imed (state when you hope to achieve it).

Take your vision (step 1) and put a deadline to it. ot to keep you bound or trapped, but rather **to guide your subconscious mind as it steers you towards your desired goal.** This is where cybernetics comes into play. The principle of the guided missile operates in your mind as well. You programme the target (your SMART goal), and your mind gets to work steering you towards it.

Your course won't be a straight line (it never is), but it will see that you end up on target, as long as the target is clearly defined (steps 1 & 4) and kept at the forefront of your consciousness at all times (steps 2 & 3).

So, no matter what may be said about goal-setting, the truth remains that it works, if you work it right.

7. **Plan and Take Action:** Work out a plan of action. Break down the plan into baby steps. Take a step or two each day, reminding yourself that each step is bringing you closer to your goal. Perform each act to the best of your ability, filled with faith, determination and purpose to reach your goal. Most importantly, be consistent.

Each task, **done properly**, is sure to lead you to your breakthrough. When things don't work out exactly as you wish, consider it to be feedback, learn from it, make the necessary adjustments to your plan and **keep going.**

One good thing about baby steps is that **they keep you from procrastinating** (you will learn more ways to overcome this deadly habit, later on in the book). They make the task at hand look easily achievable. That makes you more likely to get on with it. And for each baby step you complete, you experience the joy, and increased confidence, of success. This motivates you to take the next step, and your successes continue piling up and adding up until your vision is manifested.

So you see, positive thinking is not enough. Affirming, believing, imagining and all the rest are not enough without this one thing: **appropriate action**. It makes everything click into place. The other things pretty much set you up to perform the appropriate action.

So grab a sheet of paper and a pen. Find a quiet spot where you won't get distracted. Now begin to brainstorm (you could do this with a trusted friend, if you wish.). Write down as many ideas of possible action to take as you can think of. Keep your copy of your Vision in front of you at all times, for that will make it easier for you to recognise the pieces of the puzzle, so to speak.

Take one action step as soon as possible after your brainstorming session. Then another, and another.

8. **Persistence:** Do not give up until you have achieved what you desire. In the course of things, be willing to change any part of your plan which turns out not to work, and try something else. Thomas Edison did not give up in his quest to invent the light bulb, even though he'd 'failed' 10,000 times. Now that's persistence! See every 'failure' as a stepping-stone to success and as a temporary set back. It's been said that there's no such thing as failure, only feedback. Learn from it and push on towards your goal.

Acknowledge that it's not always going to be easy to do what you need to do. Many times you may not feel like waking up to do that workout. You may not feel like phoning that prospect or following up on that prospect. You may not feel like kissing and making up with your lover. But remember the desired result. Remember your design. Keep your eyes (and mind) on it and persist in doing what you need to do.

Refuse to give up or give in to quick-fixes or apparently easy ways out. Think long term.

Your goal is truly worth all the effort and persistence it takes.

9. **Gratitude:** Maintain an attitude of gratitude, knowing that your dream is about to become a reality. Refuse to grumble when circumstances look contrary. Refuse to complain. Be grateful for where you are now, and for where you are headed. Look around for things to be grateful for. You'll be surprised to find quite a few.

An amazing thing happens when you offer up praise and gratitude for the things happening in your life. An equal and opposite-in-direction reaction is set up. Or as the psalmist says, 'when praises go up, the blessings come down'.

Here's something else about gratitude: when you are giving thanks for something, your mind is focusing on that thing, right? And what happens to what you focus on? It expands. You get more of the same. So gratitude is a powerful mechanism of activating the Law of Attraction into your life. It's one of Seven Natural Laws.

When things look like they're going wrong, that's when you need to offer even more gratitude: believe there's good in everything, and offer gratitude **even when the good is not apparent to you.** As you persist in giving thanks, the good will become apparent, and you will attract more of it into your life.

Be serious and deliberate about your gratitude – it is one of the most underutilized, yet powerful success tools in any arsenal. You can't be depressed with an attitude of gratitude. You can't feel upset for long when you choose to maintain an attitude of gratitude. Gratitude is an excellent state to be in, conducive for creativity, productivity, success.

10. **Become a giver.** In your relationships, always think in terms of what you can do for the other person. What goes round, comes round. After all, whatever dreams you have, they most likely involve interacting with other people. Be kind and generous to all; you never know where your breakthrough will come from.

It's the old Law of Reciprocity at work: give and you will be given. **It's not your place to be concerned about who will give to you.** Just focus on giving to others, and God will sort you out.

In business, don't be afraid to give some of your best material away for free. Ask Seth Godin what good it's done him to do just this. When you give away quality material, God rewards you by making you able to produce more quality material, which you can then sell for a good price. You see, in giving away high-valued material, prospects will be thinking 'if this is what she's giving away for free, imagine what her paid stuff is like!', and they'll happily pay you what you ask when you do ask.

You can never outgive God. So be free in your giving. Don't hold back and He won't hold back from you, PLUS you'll never be wanting for anything. That's the system in place to provide for all creation. Plug into it and reap.

11. **Be in the know:** Find out everything you can about your situation/goal. Read books, listen to tapes, and talk to experts, whatever it takes. This will help you make wise decisions and keep you confident as you go along.

   Devote at least 15 minutes each day to studying personal development material, and at least another 15 minutes each day to studying material from your industry. This will keep you at the top of your game, as the mediocre masses don't bother to do so. Obviously the more time you spend studying the better you become, sooner.

   Readers are Leaders.
   Learners are Earners.

   As Bob Proctor puts it, 'join the 6 a.m. club' - wake up an hour earlier and get some reading done. It can only serve you well.

   So there you have it. If you act on these principles **consistently**, you WILL succeed in any endeavour.

Don't just take my word for it though. Prove it yourself by actually applying it to your life situation.

Knowledge is not powerful until you act on what you know. Think about that. Better yet, act on it! You'll be glad you did.

EXERCISE

- GAP

- Read through this chapter again.

- Turn each principle into a heading and write a list of the headings you see.

- Which one of those areas do you need most help improving?

- Write down what you can do to improve in the area you've selected.

- What new action or step will you take today, based on what you've read in this chapter?

NOTES

"Success depends upon previous preparation, and without such preparation there is sure to be failure."
Confucius

DAY 3
SUCCESS PRIMERS: HABITS

Every woman wants to be able to do or have whatever she desires in life. Some women succeed in doing so while others do not. What is the difference between these groups of women?

The difference is in the way the successful women are, and the way they do things. In the course of my research into habits of success since 1995, I have noticed some common themes occurring in the lives of successful women.

In order to have what you want, you have to be a certain type of person who does things in a certain way. The order is Be->Do->Have.

Today you will learn about the 'starter' information you need to get into the right frame of mind for achieving success in any project you undertake from now on.

If you take this information on board, you **will** effectively be setting yourself up to succeed in life.

All the knowledge and tools in the world are useless unless you apply them. Be a doer of the word, not a hearer (or reader) only.

What challenge are you facing right now?
- Do you want to lose weight?
- Find a better paying job?
- Start your own business?
- Get more customers/clients for your existing business?
- Find a life partner?
- Learn a new language or musical instrument?
- Do you want to be financially independent?
- Learn how to manage your emotions instead of letting them control you?
- Enjoy healthy and happy relationships?
- Manage your time better?
- Write a book?

Whatever you want to do, there are some **basic principles** you need to apply in order to do it successfully.

Success is not a destination. It is a way of life that you can choose. It is also a predictable way of doing things. It's not about luck. However you define success is personal to you, and it is up to you to achieve it for yourself. No one else can do it for you.

Over the next few days we will explore five basic 'primers' for your success. These primers position you so that your success becomes inevitable.

The journey of success you are about to embark on will not always be easy. However, the hard times **will** pass. They are temporary. Remember this, for when you do, you will rise above whatever difficulties you face and come out stronger.

Assess your current situation and decide which area of your life you want to work on first.

You can choose more than one area to work on but no more than three at a time. That way you won't feel overwhelmed by what you need to do.

Today you will learn about the first Success Primer.

Success Primer #1: HABITS OF SUCCESS

A habit is something you do almost automatically, because you've done it for so long. When you repeatedly do something, it becomes second nature to you. It becomes a habit.

If you desire to succeed in any area of your life, you must **form good habits, and then 'become their slave'** (as Og Mandino put it in his classic 'The Greatest Salesman in the World').

Before You Can Form Habits To Help You Achieve Success, You Must Define Success

First thing you need to do is decide what success means to you. Define success for yourself, not by other people's standards. **Then form habits that support your definition.** I once read of a man who defined success as earning $5 million annually. Since he was earning 'just' $2 million, he considered himself a failure and was very stressed out.

On the other hand there was a man who considered himself to be successful every day he woke up 'above ground'. All this guy had to do was wake up alive and he was celebrating his success for the day! Can you imagine how resourceful he must feel every day?

Your personal definition of success can put you in a frame of mind that allows you to achieve it easily. Or it can stress you out so much it actually hinders you from achieving it.

How would you define success? Choose a definition that will make it easy for you because success breeds more success. Here are some questions to help you figure out what it means to you. Answer them truthfully. Remember, this is your life we're talking about, not a dress rehearsal.

Which area of your life would you like to succeed in?

For each area of life you choose, describe how it would feel to be successful. How would it look, smell, taste even (!), sound? Picture it as clearly as you can. What do you see?

Write this down.

It's important for you to know the outcome you desire. That way you will be alert to opportunities to help you get it.

Once you know your desired outcome in a certain area of your life, you need to form habits that will help you achieve it.

Let's now go on to examine...

How To Form Habits of Success

A habit is a person's way of doing things. Habits are usually automatic - you don't think about what you're doing at the time. You have programmed yourself (knowingly or not) to think and act in a specific way in response to specific stimuli.

Examples of habits include lighting a cigarette when you're under stress, or brushing your teeth just before you go to bed every night. What are some of your habits?

Not all habits are useful or profitable.

Some are self-destructive (like smoking), yet hard to stop because you have ingrained those patterns of behaviour so deeply in your brain by repeating them (though in smoking there's the added effect of the addictive nature of nicotine...but that's outside the scope of this book).

Here is a simple exercise for you to do regarding bad habits. Play with me here.

Some habits are good (like brushing your teeth or exercising regularly). These are the ones you want to continue, since they have benefits to you in both the short and long term.

If you feel overwhelmed by your bad habits, relax. Nobody expects you to change all of them at once. Little steps will get you where you eventually want to be. Instead of getting overwhelmed by the big picture, form 'baby step' habits that make the journey achievable and fun.

Celebrate every successful 'baby step'. That way you will stay motivated to keep pushing on.

Frame it in positive language

If you want to change a bad habit, think in terms of what alternative good habit you want to cultivate. The human mind can only process information when it is presented to it in positive language.

Try it for yourself: if I tell you 'Don't think about a red elephant', what is the first thing you'll think of? That's right - a red elephant! Your mind read that instruction as 'think of a red elephant' and that's exactly what you did. It tends to drop words like 'not', 'don't' and other negative words from the instructions it receives. Put another way: you can't not think about something without first thinking about it.

Your mind is where your automatic behaviour comes from. You want to give it the right instructions in a language that enables it to bring about the result you desire, which in this case is to cultivate a good habit.

To get your mind to help you succeed in changing that undesirable habit, state your desire positively any time you think about it or talk about it. And think about it often. You can condition yourself to form a new habit by repeatedly thinking and talking about it. This will make it easy for you to perform the new behaviour until it becomes automatic.

For example, let's say you want to stop smoking as a reaction to feeling stressed. Instead of stating that intention as 'I will not smoke when I'm stressed' (which your mind will read as 'I will smoke when I'm stressed' - making you want to do just that!), think of a positive way to state it, such as 'I will deal with my stress by running round the block' or some such statement.

What you focus on expands, so choose to focus on the actual outcome you seek, as opposed to focusing on the outcome you're trying to stop.

The point is to <u>state your intention in terms of what you want to do</u>, and not in terms of what you don't want to do.

So now that you know what outcome you desire in a particular area of your life, decide the supportive habit(s) you need to form to make it happen.

What Makes Up A Habit?

According to Steven Covey in his book 'The 7 Habits of Highly Effective People', every habit has the following components:

- Knowledge and Attitude - what the behaviour entails. Why you need to do it. Be in the know about it, and be willing to continue learning about it. How you think about it.

- Skill - how to do what you want to do.

- Desire - you must actually want to do it.

- In addition, I believe that to form a habit, you also need

- Persistence - the ability to stick to the process and hang in there until you achieve your target.

"We are what we repeatedly do. Excellence then, is not an act, but a habit."
Aristotle

Knowledge and Attitude

What do you want to do? If you want to get fitter and healthier, for instance, what does that mean you want to do? What exactly do you understand by the terms 'fitter and healthier' (or whatever terms you've used to describe your desire)?

Why do you want to do it? What's in it for you, what do you stand to gain from becoming fit and healthy (or whatever goal you have chosen)? If you think of enough reasons to do it you will have no problem figuring out 'how' to do it.

That's one benefit of today's exercise (see below). It helps you find out why you do the things you do (what's in it for you), and why you want to change a certain behaviour pattern (what it's costing you).

So decide exactly what you want to do. Rephrase your bad habits into positive alternatives. Pick one to three habits to cultivate at this time.

To help you choose which habit to work on, refer to today's exercise. Pick one to three areas of your life to work on for the next couple of months.

For each area

- Describe a '10' state of things

- Decide why you want to reach that score of '10'

- Note which bad habits are keeping you from '10'.

- Decide which good habit would help you reach a score of 10. What would you have to do differently in order to achieve a '10'?

What can you start doing today, to get you closer to a '10'?

Think of as many reasons for forming this good habit as possible, and write them down. List all the good things (payoffs) you'll get as a result of doing it, and also list all the bad things (costs) that'll happen if you don't do it.

You might end up having two similar lists at the end of today but that's okay. You're **reconditioning your mind** to get used to the new pattern you're forming, so the more often you feed it with the right information, the better.

Repetition is the mother of skill and learning, after all. It also happens to be the key to mastering good habits.

Continue learning about your new habits and your desired state of affairs ('10' on the list of areas). Don't just learn this stuff though.

I'll harp on this quite a bit, because I'm amazed at how many women know what to do to make their lives better, yet don't do it. Matter of fact, 80% of the women who read this book will NOT act on this information. They are the same people who read all the books, attend all the courses and seminars, come home but take no action.

These same women are the ones who complain that 'all this self-help stuff doesn't work'. Go figure.

Now that you know what you want to do, you need to know 'how' to do it. Which brings us to the next ingredient of successful habit-forming....

Skill
Continuing from our previous example, if you want to get fit and healthy, how are you going to do it? What do you need to do (or stop doing) in order to become that way? What are you doing now that's stopping

you from being fit and healthy? How can you change such destructive behaviour? What can you replace it with?

These are the sorts of questions you need to ask yourself in order to get you started in your new habit.

For each area of your life that you've chosen to work on, find out and write down how you will achieve your desired goals. Will you need any outside help? Write it down. Which other resources will you need?

Write down how you are going to do what you want to do and what it'll take for you to achieve it. If you start to feel discouraged, look through your lists of costs and pay-offs (also known as 'pain and pleasure').

Remind yourself of the benefits in store for you if you stay on track and the bad stuff in store for you if you don't stay on track. That should motivate you quite a bit.

Writing things down makes you clear on what you need to do. It also keeps you focused and motivated, which is good when you're forming a habit.

So get ready to do a lot more writing in the weeks to come! It's a fun thing to do: you're literally writing your future!

The next ingredient you need to successfully form a habit is…

Desire
You must truly want the end result you say you want. Not to be like the Joneses or to impress anyone else, but to bring you personal fulfilment and satisfaction.

If you do not really want something, you won't have any incentive to keep pressing on towards your goal during tough times, and believe me there will be tough times – times when you just don't feel like doing what you should, or when people around you are doing something different and you feel alone in your quest.

What helps during times such as these is to remember what your desire is, and remember that what you're doing is bringing you closer to it.

It should be a true desire - not 'I should want this', but 'I really want this'. Make sure you really want your stated end result and you will find it easy to form the right habits to help you get it.

Persistence
For any new behaviour to become automatic, you need to persist in doing it. There's no other way to condition your mind to accept the new behaviour. Repeat it until it becomes second nature to you.

Stick to it. You owe it to yourself to enjoy the benefits of a successful lifestyle.

You won't always feel like doing things in the new way you've chosen, but decide to continue doing so anyway. This is one key that separates successful people from failures. Because it is easier to give up than to persist, people who fail tend to give up. Successful people on the other hand, persist in doing what they are doing (whether or not they enjoy the activity) because they realise it's the only way they will get what they want.

SUMMARY

Today we looked at how to form habits that lead to success.

We first defined the word 'habit'. Then you did the exercise on the costs and benefits of your current bad habits.

Finally we discussed how to form a habit. I also shared a couple of examples from my experience to show you how to apply what you've read.
I will now share an example from my life to illustrate how to apply these principles practically.

WORTH THE WEIGHT?

I was overweight after having my baby back in 2000. I wanted to shed the excess baggage but I also wanted to sit around and not do any exercise. When I realised that my habits were contradictory to my desired outcome, I decided to do something about it.

I did everything I've talked about above, starting with naming my intention positively ('I intend to get fitter, trimmer, healthier'). I identified the habits that were preventing me from being that way (not exercising, eating when not hungry). I listed the costs (fat, uncomfortable slob) and pay-offs (fun to slouch around and pig out while watching a movie) of those bad habits.

Then I rephrased the bad habits into new ones I needed to form (start exercising, eat only when hungry). I wrote the benefits I would derive from these new habits (stronger, leaner, healthier, better looking body, fat-burning machine, more energy and drive etc).

I knew I needed to exercise, so I researched to find out the right exercise programme for me; I also studied about food, nutrition and similar topics (gaining knowledge). The more I learned, the more motivated I was to stick to my new behaviour pattern.

Today, although I have successfully stuck to an exercise regime and healthy eating pattern, I continue to learn about them, keep myself up to date on research findings and tweak my programme accordingly.

From my research, I found out how to do the exercises properly then turned that into a skill by actually doing them.

My desire to remain fit and healthy is strong as ever, and what motivates me these days is the positive results of my efforts, namely, more strength and fitness, less weight, increased confidence and general feeling of well-being.

This is also why health, fitness, wellness, nutrition are topics I'm passionate about helping you with: your life improves in so many tremendous ways when you treat your body the right way in terms of nourishment and physical activity...see 'Inspirational Blueprints For Health and Wellness' for more on this.)

Now go ahead and work through today's exercise.

EXERCISE

The main aim of this exercise is to make you AWARE of the thoughts and motivation behind your bad habit patterns. Awareness is usually the first step if you want to change any behaviour.

Another aim is for you to discover the price you're paying for continuing those bad habits.

- GAP

- List your bad habits.

- Write them down on a blank sheet of paper.

- For each habit, write down the pay-offs you're getting by continuing in them. 'Pay-offs?' I hear you ask. Yes, pay-offs. One fact of human nature is that we generally do something if there's some (perceived) good in it for us. Examples of pay-offs - 'It makes me feel good' or 'my friends accept me more when I do it', or 'it makes me feel confident and in control'. Notice that the pay-offs are 'good feelings'. We do things that make us feel good.

- Next, write down what it's costing you to continue your habit. Examples of costs - 'It's draining me financially', or 'It will make me ill if I continue', 'My breath stinks and my teeth look awful because I smoke'

- What do you notice about your bad habits after doing this exercise?

- How do you feel about each one now? Many people get motivated to change simply by doing this exercise. That's a good first step.

NOTES

"First we make our habits, then our habits make us"
Spanish proverb

DAY 4
SUCCESS PRIMERS: VALUES

"It's not hard to make decisions when you know what your values are."
Roy Disney

What Are Values?

Our values are those things that are very important to us. They define who we are. They form a framework within which we operate.

Values are personal to each individual. Stephen King values his writing so highly that he's committed to writing 2000 words each day, come what may.

One of Oprah's values is reading, so she has a lot of books in her home, including a huge stack in her bathroom!

I value my family life, so I have decided to build a career around it, instead of living the other way round.

Notice how our values determine our actions. Whether or not we are aware of our values, they are the basis for our behaviour. When our actions are out of line with our values, we feel frustrated and dissatisfied. When our actions line up with our values, though, we feel tremendous peace, and in that state are more likely to be successful in what we do.

When Your Actions Don't Line Up With Your Values

Does this happen to you or someone you know: you want to spend more time with your family but you 'have' to stay back at work and finish your project - you thus feel frustrated (which frustration you unwittingly take back home with you and unleash on the very ones you wanted to spend more time with!); or you want to eat healthy and nutritious meals but you're too busy to prepare them so you order some greasy fast food instead - and end up feeling guilty and a failure, because you feel you've messed up.

Or how about this scenario? You believe you should be honest in your business dealings but your boss gets you to 'bend the truth a little' in order to please a customer.

Think of other times that you've been frustrated with your situation. Or felt guilty. What's happening in each example above is that you are violating your values.

Each time that happens, you feel horrible, don't you? And when you feel horrible about yourself or your situation you become unable to be resourceful, and you repel success in that state.

The Danger of Violating Your Values

When your goals and actions are out of line with your values, you suffer in many ways, sometimes without knowing why.

Here are a couple of ways; some have been alluded to already:

- You feel frustrated. As a result of this frustration you become stressed. The bad thing about this is that you may take out your frustration on the wrong person, since you're not aware of its true source. This can hurt your relationship with that person, as you can imagine.

- When your values are incongruent with your actions, you are more likely to fail in those actions because you are in an unresourceful state. On the other hand, when they line up perfectly, you become unstoppable. Remember Stephen King? His actions (writing 2000 words daily) perfectly match his values (good writing) and the results are clear for all to see.

- Guilt and damage to your self-esteem: you feel you've let yourself down when you do something that violates your values. It's a most unpleasant feeling, this one.

The Benefits of Honouring Your Values

When your goals and actions match your values, you benefit greatly.

- Success comes naturally and more easily to you. If you value your health and fitness, and act accordingly (eat healthily and exercise regularly), you will succeed in becoming fit and healthy. If you value family relationships, and you therefore put your work, career or business in its right place, you will be rewarded with a healthy, happy family relationship.

The benefits of honouring your values are priceless.

- You are a lot more focused when your goals and actions are congruent with your values. This type of focus makes success inevitable.

What Are YOUR Values?

By now you probably understand how important values are. It's time for you to wake up and take stock of your own values. What are they? Remember, awareness is the first step towards any change or improvement.

Let's find out what your values are. You want to know them so that you can begin to align your goals and actions accordingly, deliberately.

In today's exercise you will discover what your true values are.

Your next step will then be to make sure your goals and actions line up with them. Starting NOW!

What do you want to achieve? Business success? Health and fitness? Career success? Sound relationships?

Begin to align your goals and actions with your values in each area. I tell you, nothing will stand in your way of achieving outstanding success in any of those areas when you do!

SUMMARY

In this chapter you have learned about values, what they are and why you need to (a) be aware of yours and (b) make your goals and actions congruent with them.

This stuff is really powerful. I speak from experience.

Do the following exercise. You WILL see results when you apply these principles to your life. And I want to hear all about your great results when they start happening!

EXERCISE

GAP. Make a list of the top five most important things in your life. Arrange them in order of priority, with the most important one at the top of the list.

Examples from my clients have included:
- Love
- Financial independence
- Integrity
- Success
- Relationships
- Family
- Career
- Spirituality

I have included those examples to give you an idea of what values are.

What are yours? They may or may not be on the list, it doesn't matter. Your values are personal to you.

As you can imagine, if integrity (for example) is one of your values, and your job involves actions that are dishonest, no matter how highly paid you are, you will be dissatisfied in that job. You probably won't be doing well in it either.

~~FOOD FOR THOUGHT~~

Take a minute and look back in your life: those times you've struggled with some issue or other (and who hasn't at some point?), and felt frustrated that things weren't going your way.

Which of your values do you think you were violating at that time?

NOTES

DAY 5
SUCCESS PRIMERS: RESPONSIBILITY

"No one can make you jealous, angry, vengeful, or greedy - unless you let him."
Napoleon Hill

You are responsible for the outcome of your life.
You are responsible for your future.

The moment you accept this truth, you empower yourself to change things that aren't working in your life.

There are certain things you can't control or do anything about, but there are many things in your life that you **can** control.

Things such as your moods, emotions, attitudes, your thoughts, your words, your responses, your actions, your choices and decisions - these are all under your influence.

Your life today is the result of how you have handled the things under your control, whether or not you have been aware of them.

It is very easy to blame others for things ('she made me so angry, I had to say what I did' or 'I'm a woman, so my chances in this career are limited' or 'the weather was bad so I could not attend that training course').

But blaming others for things puts them in control of your life, and makes you a victim.

Acknowledge and accept responsibility for every aspect of your life, and you will experience a freedom and power that enables you to pursue your goals and dreams with vigour.

What about the things in your life that you can't control? Such as other people's behaviour, the current situation in the Middle East, or the weather?

What should you do about them? The only thing you can do about such things is to change the way you see them. Change the way you think about them.

> Change the way you think about the things you can't do anything about.

Focus your attention on the things you can do something about. The things you focus your attention on expand in your life. This means that they affect you in more ways than you may be aware of.

Think about it: if you spend time thinking about things that are upsetting, how do you feel? How productive are you in that state of mind? Not very, right?

On the other hand, if you spend your time thinking of positive things, pleasant things, exciting possibilities (and life is full of these), you feel very good inside. As a result you will be more productive and resourceful, instead of being stuck in a rut.

If you spend time thinking about things you can control, you will be alert to ideas and opportunities to do something about your situation. You will be aware of chances to improve your lot.

And you will be more inclined to seize those opportunities.

It pays to focus on controlling the things you can. You can control your thoughts. You can control your words and actions. Take responsibility for them and refuse to give up control to outside forces.

It's your life and you owe it to yourself to direct it the way you want it to go.

The word 'responsibility' is a combination of two words: 'Response' and 'Ability'. You have the ability to choose your response to any situation in your life. So choose wisely.

EXERCISE

- In which areas of your life are you omitting to own responsibility? Who (or what) do you blame for the way your life is in those areas? Be truthful here – this is a personal thing, nobody else has to know your answers.

- GAP and write this down.

- Now decide to take responsibility for those areas of your life if it was up to you (and it is, most likely). How would you do things, how would you like things to turn out?

- Write this down. What do you notice?

- It's all about the way you see things, remember. So begin to see things in ways that empower you. Begin to see yourself as being in control of your life, as being responsible for your thoughts, feelings, words and actions (including the way you respond to circumstances and other people). Begin to see yourself as responsible and in control of your life.

NOTES

"The willingness to accept responsibility for one's own life is the source from which self-respect springs"
Joan Didion

DAY 6
SUCCESS PRIMERS: SELF-DISCIPLINE

"Discipline is the bridge that links your thought to its accomplishment"
Jim Rohn

The phrase 'self-discipline' makes many people shudder. Probably because it conjures negative images of pain, suffering and deprivation.

That's not what self-discipline is about. Truly applied, self-discipline is one of the most liberating forces known to man.

Self-discipline implies the use of your inherent power to keep your emotions, thoughts, and actions in check. It means **making yourself think, do and say the right things.**

To be blunt, there is no way you can consistently do the things you want to do, unless you exercise self-discipline.

Self-discipline is a powerful and very useful attitude and can become a habit with practice. It takes self-control to stay committed to any chosen course of action. Even thinking the right thoughts requires self-discipline.

But first you must realise that you do have the inherent power, you are capable of directing your thoughts, words and actions.

Unless you recognise and accept that fact, you won't see the point in making any effort.

Decide to direct your thoughts, words and actions towards whatever goal you choose. That is easier said than done, I admit, but it can be done and you can do it.

You CAN choose what you think about. So think about the things you want to be, and the things you want to do.

Think about good things, even (and most especially) when it's hard to do so. When you're going through a difficult time, tell yourself that there's good in this somewhere and be thankful for that good even when it's not yet apparent.

You attract the things you think about most of the time. That's one reason why it is vital that you monitor your thoughts.

You CAN choose your words, so choose them wisely. Words are powerful things, and have more far-reaching effects than most people know.

Your words influence the way you feel at any given time, same as your thoughts do. Words are things which have life in them. The power of death and life are in your tongue, so speak words that bring life to you and those around you.

You CAN choose your actions. Nobody can make you do anything, you know. Not really. Think about it. Bear in mind that every action you (choose to) do, has consequences for which you are responsible (see previous chapter).

Commit today to practise self-control over your thoughts, words and actions, and then DECIDE to honour your commitments to yourself. Whatever you decide to do, do it whether or not you feel like doing it. This is one thing that differentiates winners from losers in life.

Be a winner. Practise daily discipline until it's a habit. This exercise below will help you.

EXERCISE

Start to keep track of the thoughts that occupy your mind.

- GAP.

- In a notebook, draw a line and form two columns, one with the heading 'Positive/good thoughts' and the other with the heading 'Negative/bad thoughts'.

- Fill in the columns as often as you are aware of your thoughts.

- This will make you aware of your predominant thought pattern.

- Do this exercise daily for a week.

Once you become aware of your thought patterns, you can change them by replacing the negative ones with corresponding positive ones.

You must then persist in holding only the positive, empowering thoughts at all times, in your mind regardless of outward appearances.

When you master disciplining your thoughts you will find it easy to apply discipline to your words and actions as well.

NOTES

"It was character that got us out of bed, commitment that moved us into action, and discipline that enabled us to follow through."
Zig Ziglar

DAY 7
SUCCESS PRIMERS: DETERMINATION

"The difference between the impossible and the possible lies in a person's determination."
Tommy Lasorda

To achieve long-term success in any venture, you must be determined to succeed.

It helps if your goal is something you are actually interested in accomplishing. It has to be YOUR goal, no one else's.

It also helps if you want to accomplish it for the right reasons, and if those reasons agree with your values (notice how these primers all tie in together). Once your 'why' for doing something is big enough and important enough to you, once you realise that you do not wish to pay the price for not accomplishing it, you will be determined to do what it takes to get you there.

When you are determined to do something, your chances of succeeding in that thing are very high.

The great thing about determination is that it's a choice you make. That's right, like many things in life, you can choose to be determined about your goals or not.

As David Livingstone said, **'I determined never to stop until I had come to the end and achieved my purpose.'**

Notice that he purposely determined to keep pressing on until he'd achieved his purpose.

The same thing has to apply to you.

I like the way Benjamin Disraeli put it here: **"Nothing can resist the human will that will stake even its existence on its stated purpose."**

But you have to state your purpose first. Which you've done, haven't you? Good. Glad to know you're among the active 20% who achieve results that the inactive 80% only dream about.

Being determined implies you have acknowledged that things won't always be rosy on this journey. It also implies that you've accepted this fact and are prepared (mentally at least) to face and surmount obstacles as they come. In other words, you have 'counted the cost' and are willing to pay the price to attain your objective.

Be determined now, dear reader. Whatever you want to achieve is truly within your grasp. Refuse to get distracted or discouraged. Stay determined and you will succeed.

EXERCISE

- GAP.

- Think of one goal you would like to achieve.

- How does it make you feel? Think about how your life will be when you've accomplished it. Describe the picture that comes to your mind (yes, write it down - you should know by now that you need to read this book with pen and paper handy).

- How do you feel about the picture you see in your mind?

- Does it stimulate, challenge and inspire you? Does it make you want to get started on the journey already?

- If it doesn't, rewrite your goal until it does.

- Now look at your 're-charged' goal. It should make you feel like you really want to go for it.

- Whether or not you feel like it though (and chances are that your inner 'nasty voice' is telling you reasons why you shouldn't even dream of reaching for that goal), once you are sure that this is something you want, consciously determine in your heart that you'll get it.

- Write down your decision. It should look something like this:

- "I am determined to do whatever is necessary and appropriate in order to (release five kilos of unwanted fat in the next six weeks.)"

- Replace the words in bracket above with your goal, being sure to include the time frame you intend to achieve it in. Replacing the words 'am determined' with the word 'will', makes the statement more powerful and also helps you stay determined to achieve what you want.

- Even better is to replace it with the word 'am' – this makes your subconscious get into 'present mode' and cause you to begin doing things now, towards your goal. If you leave the statement with 'will', then your mental programming remains in 'future mode', always getting there but never quite arriving.

- When you replace it with the word 'am' it reads like this: 'I am achieving my goal of (releasing five kilos of unwanted fat from my body over the next six weeks).

- You get the idea. You will learn more about affirmations later but the above example is a good jump-start for you.

- Affirm your determination several times each day, at least twice a day (first thing in the morning and last thing at night).

- This conscious decision will come in very handy when things seem particularly difficult.

NOTES

"Failure will never overtake me if my determination to succeed is strong enough"
Og Mandino

DAY 8
USE YOUR IMAGINATION TO SUCCEED

"Your imagination is there to help you create the life you want in your mind before you create it physically."
Dr Kem Thompson

You were created with the power to live a truly abundant life if you chose to. Right now, you have all you need to become who you want to be, to do what you want to do and to have what you want to have.

The trouble is you may be unaware of how to harness this power. What's the point of having a million dollars in a safe if you don't know the combination to unlock it?

The best things in life are usually free. The truth is free, and having laid the foundation in the preceding chapters, you will now begin a journey of discovery of some powerful truths which (when you ACT ON THEM) will transform you into the great woman you are destined to be.

What do you want? I mean, what do you really, really want? Don't ever let anyone steal your dreams from you. They (your dreams) are there for a reason.

Here's a 'secret' for you: The fact that you want something is proof that you can obtain it. The very desire in you to be, do or have something is evidence that you've got what it takes to make it happen. Please stop right there and chew on that statement for a bit. When you make this truth your own, dream-stealers will never stand in your way again.

Whatever you want, it is possible for you to have. Or as Napoleon Hill put it, **'what the human mind can conceive and believe, the human mind can achieve'.** Don't let anyone tell you different.

You are no different from all the great achievers who have ever lived. You have a mind, the same as they did (and do). You may differ from them though in the way you use your mind.

Which brings me to the very first step you need to take in order to get what you want in life. Did you answer the question I asked you earlier: what do you want?

Let me expand it a bit:
- Who do you want to become? (which implies 'that you're not')
- What do you want to do in your life? (..'that you're not doing?')
- What do you want to have? (...'that you don't have?')

Don't answer the above questions in a hurry. Spend some time thinking about them before you answer. I don't want you to limit your thinking in any way.

Answer those questions as if you had no limitations whatsoever (money, time etc).

To expand your thinking even further, let's add this little phrase to the above questions:

If you could have, be or do anything at all without any limitations or obstacles...

What would you be?
What would you do?
What would you have?

Write down the answers to these questions. Let your imagination roam free. That's what it's there for: to help you visualise what you want. To help you create the life you want in your mind before you create it physically. It's the same way an architect designs a house before it gets built. You are the architect of your own life and your 'designing ground' is in your mind, using your imagination.

Your imagination is the workshop where you create the Blueprints for Success in your (outward) life.

There are always two creations: one invisible and intangible, the second visible and tangible.

The first step in getting what you want therefore is:

- **Know exactly what you want.** Put another way, you need to form a clear, definite, precise, mental picture (or vision) of what you want.

- **Hold this picture in your mind all the time.** Think about it often. Spend your spare time thinking about it.

God created you with the ability to imagine things. Ever wonder why? Your imagination is the workshop where you create your vision, the vision of your life. It is a true statement that 'people perish where there is no vision' (King Solomon the wise (Proverbs 29:18)).

Learn now the reason for which you were given the gift of imagination and begin today to put it to its originally intended use.

You are to use your imagination to create images of the life you want to live. It bears repeating until you can grasp the implications of this statement.

Think of the way you want your life to be. Engage all your senses in this exercise (how does it look, how does it feel, what smells and tastes are there in your life? what sounds surround you in your ideal life?). Write these down.

Come on, play along! Don't just read these words without acting on them. This is fun stuff yet it is powerful and effective.

As you write down the things you want, tell yourself **'It is possible for me to have this'** or **'I can do this'**. Say that to yourself each step of the way. This will begin to open up your mind to the great possibilities and opportunities that surround you every single day.

When you have written down your dreams, your ideal life, keep the picture at the top of your mind all the time. Think about it all the time.

Life is truly exciting when you realise that 'if it's to be, it's up to you'. If it's to be, it's up to me. Make that one of your 'success mantras'.

Then look at what you've written down again and remind yourself that 'the fact that I desire it means I have what it takes to obtain it; it means that it's possible for me to be, do and have it'.

Remember that every thing you see around you started in someone's mind. Someone was using his/her imagination well and that's how we've ended up with all the amazing facilities in the world today.

Take the very first step towards your desired destination and guard your vision very closely. You will face dream-stealers along the way but do not let them distract you from your picture.

Focus on your dream, remembering that it is possible for you to attain it and that it is up to you to do so. This is where you need to apply the 'bridge' – self-discipline - to your imagination. You need to stay focused on your desired outcome.

Now that you have written down what you want, keep that picture in your mind at all times. I cannot emphasise this point enough. If I sound repetitive, it's deliberate, for repetition is the mother of all learning.

One key to success is focus. Being focused will get you what you want faster than if you were distracted and all over the place. Being focused helps your subconscious mind co-operate with you to achieve your goals.

Dangers of losing focus:

- When you lack focus, your brain receives mixed signals and is unable to help you accomplish any one thing.

- You tend to get discouraged when you don't see the results you seek.

- You are unable to concentrate on any given task; this makes your workmanship shoddy.

- You feel confused.

- You become forgetful. You forget your purpose.

- You feel frustrated.

- Ultimately you don't get what you want. You fail.

Benefits of focusing on what you want:
- What you focus on expands; you attract the things you think about most of the time. Your life today is the result of the dominant thoughts that have occupied your mind over the years. Therefore to create a better future, focus on your mental image of that future.

- You become more confident that you'll get it.

- Your brain continues to work even while you're asleep, to find ways for you to accomplish your goals.

- You remain motivated to keep pushing on.

- Obstacles don't faze you. Instead they lessen in significance when compared to your picture.

- You become more alert to opportunities that move you towards your target.

- You are less prone to distractions.

- You feel happy inside.

- Focusing on your goal puts you in the right frame of mind to achieve it.

- Ultimately you get what you want. You succeed.

Having said all that, I have to warn you that keeping your mind on the things you want is one of the most difficult things you will ever have to do.

This is because all around you there are things and people screaming for your attention. The media alone is doing all it can to get you to focus on their message. These people generally don't care about your personal goals and helping you achieve them. They only care about their own goals. So you must focus on your goal until it is your dominant thought.

You can do it. Decide today to take control of your thoughts and choose what you think about carefully. Every time you find yourself thinking something different to what you want, stop immediately and change back to thinking about what you want. With determination, you will succeed.

Make a conscious effort in this area every day.

This includes thinking about your current reality. Thinking about the way things are right now is not going to change anything. However, thinking about the way you want things to be WILL change things if you hold fast to that line of thought. This is known as concentrated thinking or simply 'focus'

The exercise below will show you exactly **how** to practise concentrated thought – how to focus on what you want. Do it and reap the benefits.

I leave you with this sobering verse from the Book of Proverbs and a related thought: ***"Guard your heart <u>diligently</u> for from it are the issues of life."***

In other words, the very essence of your life depends on the thoughts you hold in your mind, so protect your mind (heart) seriously. Do not watch programmes or listen to things and people who pollute your mind with doubt and scepticism.

Only mix with people, read books, watch programmes or listen to things that strengthen your resolve to succeed in life.

EXERCISE

- GAP (if you haven't done so already)

- Write down what you desire in every area of your life.

- As you write each desire, tell yourself 'This is possible for me', 'I can do this' and 'If it's to be, it's up to me'

- Look at your list first thing in the morning and last thing at night. Look at your list during your spare moments each day.

- Each time you look at your list, tell yourself 'This is possible for me', 'I can do this' and 'If it's to be, it's up to me'.

Think about what you want all the time.

Remember, 'As a (wo)man thinketh, so is (s)he'.

NOTES

*"Let your imagination release your
imprisoned possibilities."
Robert H Schuller*

DAY 9
THE POWER OF YOUR BELIEFS

"Be not afraid of life. Believe that life is worth living and your belief will help create the fact."
William James

Before you can do what you need to do in order to reach your goals, you must believe on some level that you will make it. If you don't believe that you will achieve your ambition, you won't be motivated to take any steps towards it. Makes sense, doesn't it?

Just what are beliefs anyway?

Beliefs are thoughts which you hold to be true. This means that of themselves, beliefs are neither true or false. They just are. You are the one to decide whether a thought is true or not. You can choose to believe something or to doubt it. You can also change a belief if you find that it's holding you back from doing what you want to do.

Isn't it amazing? The power to succeed is yours by choice. Every one of us has beliefs that empower us to do great things as well as beliefs that limit us from achieving our true potential. The difference is that some people are aware of their limiting beliefs and take action to change them, while others are either unaware of their limiting beliefs, don't know how to change them or are just too plain lazy to change them. Which group describes you?

Limiting beliefs often include the phrase 'I can't' or 'I'm not' and include things such as 'I can't do anything worthwhile because I didn't go to school' or 'I can't be good at this because I'm not experienced enough' or ' I'll never get promoted because of my race' or 'I'm not pretty enough to get a date'. Ever had thoughts like those? Ever made excuses for not doing something?

Limiting beliefs let you have excuses for not going for your goals.

What effect do such thoughts have on your behaviour and feelings? Think about it. For one thing, they stop you from enjoying life. And of course they leave you with a low self-esteem.

What if you changed your limiting beliefs to empowering ones like these: 'I can learn anything I choose to and be good at it' or 'this is a good opportunity for me to gain the experience I want' or 'I'll be the best at my job and get promoted, regardless of my race - as a matter of fact, I'll be a pace-setter for others like me' or 'I am beautiful' or 'I'm all that and I love myself as I am!' or ' I thrive on challenges!'

How would those beliefs affect your behaviour? They are called 'empowering' for a reason, you know. You bet they'll get you up and raring to go for whatever project you have at hand. They will also leave you feeling confident.

When you believe you can do something, your mind finds ways for you to do it. As David J. Schwartz said in his classic 'The Magic of Thinking Big', 'believing a solution paves the way to the solution.'

One of my clients had major limiting beliefs, which were keeping her stuck in a job she hated, living a life she hated. Her beliefs included 'I've failed so many times before, I'm just no good at anything' and 'I'm never going to be good at what I do, that's why nobody will offer me a good job.' She also believed 'I can't even have a lasting relationship because I'm not worth it'.

As a result of such a mindset, she kept applying for (and getting) low-paying jobs that she hated. Notice how her beliefs determined her actions and results. Her life was such a wreck, she was crying for most of our first session.

After a few sessions working on her beliefs, she adopted a new set of empowering beliefs to guide her life.

The change in her attitude and approach to life was quite dramatic. She became confident in her abilities and unique qualities, started applying for jobs that were commensurate with her skills and experience and was offered one that she wanted. Today she is a confident young woman, rising in a field she used to dream about. And she is now in a stable relationship with a man she loves. Empowering beliefs make you attractive, see.

Your beliefs will make or break you in life. Doesn't it make sense to hold fast to beliefs that support your goals and dreams? One of my core beliefs is that 'Where there is a will to do something, there's always a way to do it'. With that belief, I keep my eyes open for ways of getting a job done. And more often than not, I find ways. You know what the Bible says, 'Seek and you shall find' - that's another belief I choose to hold, by the way.

When I wanted to attempt an academic feat that hadn't been done before back in medical school, I was plagued with thoughts like 'but nobody has ever done this before, what makes you think you will?' Now I could have let those thoughts determine my actions, but I chose to ignore those thoughts and replace them with ones like 'then I'll be the first to do it' and 'I can do all things through the power in me who gives me strength – this feat included'.

I held those thoughts until they became strong beliefs in my heart. There was no stopping me then. I excelled almost effortlessly. All because I believed I could.

You are no different.

Look back at your life right now. What beliefs can you identify that have held you back from accomplishing what you've wanted to do? What beliefs are holding you back right now? Stop and think about this then write them down.

Conversely, what beliefs were at work when you did very well at something in your life? What other empowering beliefs do you hold right now that are making things go well in certain parts of your life? Think about it. Write these down too.

Wouldn't it be great to have only empowering beliefs? The 'Rocky' movie series provides a good example of the power of your beliefs. Rocky believed he could at least go the distance with the world champion (in Rocky I). It was not easy but that was his goal, and he believed he could do it, so he went out, prepared and succeeded. The sequels show him experiencing phases of self-doubt (as we all do from time to time), but whenever he believed he could win, he acted accordingly and as a result, he won.

Notice how your beliefs always determine your actions. They literally create your reality.

How A Belief Changed The Course of A Sport

You've probably heard the story of the four-minute mile.

Briefly, before Roger Bannister ran the mile in four minutes, the general belief was that it was humanly, physiologically, impossible. Well he chose to believe differently. As a result of his belief, he set about to prepare to 'do the impossible'. And he succeeded in doing it. Since then, the general belief has changed and not only that, but the mile has been run in less than four minutes as well.

What changed? **Beliefs.** Not carved in stone, but changeable.

What if you held the belief that anything is possible for you. What if you believed that God (however you define that higher power) was on your side, willing and able to provide for your daily needs and more?

What would you do with your life? Remember, **what you believe becomes your reality.** If you believe you're a failure that will become your reality. Your life will reflect that belief.

I challenge you to change your beliefs today. Choose a set of beliefs that will empower you to take appropriate action towards your ambition in life.

Not sure what your beliefs are? Check out your daily actions, past and present. Then ask yourself why you do the things you do. The answer to that question will reveal your beliefs.

You know the old adage 'seeing is believing'? Well a more accurate adage is 'believing is seeing', because that's the way things work in life - you'd better believe it!

To learn how to change your beliefs, work through the following exercise. I've got to warn you - it's not going to be easy, but with practice and persistence **you will succeed** for it will become a habit.

EXERCISE

- GAP

- Make a list of limiting beliefs you've held in the past (such as 'I can't get a good job because I have no formal education').

- For each limiting belief, write what it has cost you to hold on to it.

- What is it going to cost you in the future if you continue to hold on to each negative belief?

- What do you want to achieve in the future?

- Write it down.

- Write what you need to believe for that to happen. What new beliefs will you hold to support your goals?

- Choose to believe this new set of thoughts. Commit to thinking your new empowering thoughts constantly until they become strong beliefs in your heart.

NOTES

"We are what we believe we are."

Benjamin N. Cardozo

DAY 10
THE ATTRACTION OF GRATITUDE

"To speak gratitude is courteous and pleasant, to enact gratitude is generous and noble, but to live gratitude is to touch Heaven."
Johannes A. Gaertner

Being grateful is one of the best things you could do for yourself in your quest for success.

Why?

Because **an attitude of gratitude keeps you in a resourceful state.** This makes you better able to come up with solutions and ideas that will help you prosper in your efforts. When you practise gratitude consistently, your brain receives signals of abundance.

This causes your subconscious brain to **attract abundance** into your life. Your subconscious now works with your conscious to bring your plans and goals to life.

On the other hand if you refuse to be thankful for what you have (even as you wait for what you want to come to you), you send messages of lack to your brain and that's what you get more of.

A more important reason for you to be actively grateful (that is, to acknowledge the good things in your life now and the good things on their way to you, and give thanks for them - even when things look contrary) is this: **a sincere outpouring of gratitude keeps you in harmony with God** (your 'Higher Power' or 'Infinite Intelligence'), who is the source of all good things.

Every cause has an equal and opposite effect (Newton's second law). When you give thanks to God, you set a cause in motion. The natural effect of that cause is an equal and opposite outpouring of blessings on your life. These blessings may come in different forms - job promotion, better relationships, lucrative business contracts, academic distinction, material possessions - you name it.

You don't even have to subscribe to any religion for this principle to work for you. It is a Universal Law. Just like gravity. **It works whether you believe it or not.** So practise daily gratitude from now on.

Another bonus you get when you make it a habit to be grateful is that you experience inner joy, which radiates as outer happiness. You become a more pleasant person to be around. You are more attractive to others. You're happy and fulfilled in life.

Because you're focused on the good things, the bad things pale in comparison and lose their power to get you down. They can't get you down any more, because with an attitude of gratitude, you're plugged into the source of all power, prosperity, health and everything that's good. Plus, you get what you focus on, so if you focus on things to be grateful for, you will attract more things to be grateful for.

Make a commitment today to be grateful every day. Can't think of anything to be grateful for? Then I ask you: if you could be grateful for anything, what would it be? Seek and you will find: **look for things to be thankful for and you will find them.**

The following exercise will help you form the habit of being grateful every day.

Do it now.

EXERCISE

- GAP

- Write down the following questions:
  'What things am I thankful for?'
  Who am I grateful to have in my life?'

- Think of as many answers as you can to each question and write them down. Remember to include your desires, dreams or goals. Be thankful for these because the One who has given you the desire has, along with it, given you thewhere withal to bring it to pass. That is something to be grateful for.

- Add answers to your list each day. Start each day by asking and answering those questions. End each day the same way. This will keep your eyes open throughout the day for things to be thankful for.

- Be serious about this. Practise these steps every day for the next seven days and let me know how you get on. Hopefully, you'll continue this exercise for the rest of your life.

How to interrupt negative thinking patterns

Here is a simple but effective way that I have used to help my clients overcome their negative thought patterns. Do it and see the results.

- Wear a rubber band around your wrist for the next 30 days. Snap the rubber band any time you catch yourself thinking something negative or limiting.

- Once you snap it, say something positive (for instance say the opposite of the negative thought you were entertaining.)

- Say it out loud.

- You may think all this stuff is 'hoaky' and not at all 'cool' but wouldn't you rather be a 'hoaky success' than a 'cool failure'?

NOTES

Being grateful attracts more things to be grateful for"
Dr Kem

DAY 11
APPROPRIATE ACTION: NOTHING HAPPENS WITHOUT IT

"Everything depends upon execution; having just a vision is no solution."
Stephen Sondheim

So far in this book, you have learned that in order to get what you want in life, you need to

- know exactly what you want and form a clear mental picture of it.

- hold that picture in your mind at all times to help you stay focused.

- believe that you can indeed attain what you want.

- be grateful for what you have and also for what you're going to have.

All the above are very important in the process of creating the life you desire. They set the creative process in motion. They cause the thing you want to start coming to you. **But they are not enough.**

That which you desire will not reach you unless you are able to receive it. **The only thing that will make you able to receive what you want** when it eventually comes is **Appropriate Action.**

'Good luck' is what happens to people who were ready to receive it when it came to them. And they got ready by being prepared. They got prepared by taking appropriate action.

What does 'Appropriate Action' mean?

It means doing the right things to get you from where you are to where you want to be.

Think about it. If you want to lose weight and get fit, you can visualise your ideal body size and believe all you want, but if you eat unhealthy foods and continue to lead a sedentary life, your dream will never come true. **Inappropriate action will move you away from your goals just as surely as inaction will.**

If you are unhappy in your job and want a better job, take the initial steps listed above in order to start the process of your ideal job coming to you. But you have to do the right thing to make you ready and able to receive your dream job when it arrives.

Appropriate action has several components. Each component should be present in anything you do.

Make every act you perform appropriate for the goal you want to achieve. If every single act you perform is done right, you have no choice but to succeed in life.

Here are **the components of 'Appropriate Action'.** For an act to be 'Appropriate',

- you must **do it with a clear idea of your desired outcome.** Do everything with a deliberate intention. Know what you expect to happen as a result of each action you take. Yes, that includes brushing your teeth. The point here is, apply this principle to even the 'small things' of your life and you'll find it easy to apply it to the 'bigger things' as well.

- you must **do it to the best of your ability.** It doesn't matter how big or small the act is. Every cause has a corresponding effect, no matter how small. Aim to set only good, excellent causes in motion in your life. That way you can only get excellent outcomes.

- you must **do it with the firm belief** that it will lead to the result you desire.

- you must **do it with a strong sense of determination.** Be determined to get what you want as a result of your actions. The Universe will pave the way for you when you act like this.

- you must **do it with total gratitude and belief that you are getting what you want.**

That should be your mindset every day, for each and every act you perform. Your life cannot help but be a success when you behave this way.

If you are in a job you don't like and you want to get a better job, get a clear mental picture of the ideal job you do want (be as precise as you can when making your picture: include exact salary expectations, working conditions, etc). Then start where you are to do your current job to the very best of your ability.

Bear in mind that you are not doing this to please your boss. You are doing this **to prepare yourself to receive** your ideal job when the opportunity comes. This way, you're telling the Universe 'yes you can entrust me with a better job. I am up to the task'. If you work with a lousy attitude and do a poor job, don't expect to be offered anything better.

This is what is meant by the concept of 'be - do - have'.

In order to have what you want, you need to become a certain type of person who does things in a way that's appropriate to the goal you want to achieve. As a result, you will have what you want.

Apply this principle to everything you want to achieve in life.

God /The Universe/Higher Power rewards appropriate action. Therefore begin today to take the right steps (no matter how small they seem) towards your goals. With a good plan in place and the right mindset, you will be unstoppable. You WILL get what you want.

Make this year different by taking appropriate action whenever you do anything. Start with the little things then move on to the big things. Remember that action is the only thing that brings you closer to your goals. You can do it, so go on and make it happen!

EXERCISE

- GAP

- Write down your major goals that you want to accomplish in the next 12 months.

- For each one, write out your plan of action to make it happen.

- Break each action plan into small baby steps. Daily activities, if you will.

- Commit to making every act you do an 'Appropriate Action'.

- Do something from your action plan NOW.

NOTES

*"Personal action is your pathway to success,
even if it is a little bit at a time!"*
Catherine Pulsifer

DAY 12
THE PROPER USE OF WILLPOWER

"You have a very powerful mind that can make anything happen as long as you keep yourself centred."
Dr. Wayne W. Dyer

Here is a general principle for you to remember: nature is friendly to you. God is for you and not against you. He has **already** given you everything you need to live the best quality of life you possibly can.

However He has also given you the power to choose how to use (or not use) the gifts you've been given.

What has this got to do with will power? Everything.

According to the principle above, your willpower has been given to you to use for your own benefit. It is there to help you achieve your heart's desire. **You are meant to use your willpower to cause your mental picture to manifest physically. Use it to make yourself focus on the the mental image of your desired outcome.**

But it won't work unless you use it properly.

What is 'Willpower' anyway? I'll give you my favourite definition.

Willpower is your ability to make yourself follow through on tasks that you set out to do.

By that definition, can you see how willpower plays a role in getting you what you want in life? You choose a goal to accomplish. You create an action plan to help you get there. You commit to follow through. Then you harness your willpower to make you follow through.

Another life principle for you to remember is this: 'Use it or lose it.'

Strengthening your willpower is not easy, but with constant practice and exercise, you will build strong, 'willpower muscles', which you can use any time you choose.

When you make yourself follow through and accomplish a goal, you feel highly satisfied and fulfilled. The whole process enriches your life. You end up feeling empowered and in control of your life.

Some people say you don't need willpower to accomplish anything. I beg to differ with them on that issue. The fact is you cannot do anything in your life without some degree of willpower. Even getting out of bed in the morning requires it.

Instead of looking for cop-outs and instant solutions, it is more profitable for you to nurture and exercise the gifts that you have already been given. Gifts like belief, willpower, choice, love, health and so on. All these gifts are there for you to live a good, long life. Use them well and you will be amazed.

Use your willpower today to achieve any or all of these:

- keep your mind focused on your goal.
- keep your thoughts in line with your goal.
- keep your actions in line with your goal.
- keep your words in line with your goal.
- persist until you succeed.
- remain consistent and not wishy-washy.
- encourage yourself when you feel down.

In short, use your willpower to stay on course for success by using it to keep your mind in the right state to achieve success.

- You want a better job? Use your willpower to maintain a good attitude in your current job while you look around.
- You want to lose weight? Use your willpower to stick to a program of regular exercise and healthy eating.
- You want a life partner? Use your willpower to keep yourself attractive inside and outside at all times.

You get the idea.

EXERCISE

- GAP.

- Write down one task you need to follow through on consistently in order to reach your goal.

- Write down what the task entails.

- Write down the answers to these questions:

    a. What do I find difficult about doing this task?
    b. Why do I find it difficult?
    c. What will my life be like one, three, five years from now if I do not perform this task?
    d. How does that future look? How does it feel?
    e. What will my life be like one, three, five years from now if I do this task?
    f. How does this alternative future look? How does it feel?
    g. Which future would I rather have?
    h. Which future would I rather work towards?
    i. What 10 benefits will I experience if I do this task consistently?
    j. What 10 disadvantages will I experience if I do not do this task consistently?

- Next time you feel tempted to neglect an activity that brings you closer to your goal, say to yourself 'I choose discipline over regret'. Say it out loud or write it down then go immediately and do that thing.

- Practise this until it becomes a habit

"When you have a number of disagreeable duties to perform, always do the most disagreeable first."
Josiah Quincy

NOTES

"It's not that some people have willpower and some don't. It's that some people are ready to change and others are not."
James Gordon

DAY 13
CHOOSE YOUR PAIN AND WORK WITH IT

"The successful person has the habit of doing the things failures don't like to do. They don't like doing them either necessarily. But their disliking is subordinated to the strength of their purpose."
E.M Gray

Every choice you make, every action you take, has prices and consequences. If you discipline yourself to do something, it seems painful at the time, but the long term result is pleasurable. If you refuse to apply discipline to getting a task done, however, it may seem pleasurable at the time, but the long term result is pain – the pain of regret.

So it looks like one way or another you've got to contend with some pain in your journey to success. It then becomes up to you to choose which pain you'd rather have – the (relatively) short term pain of discipline, or the long term pain of regret.

Just like willpower (which goes hand-in-hand with discipline), you need to practise self-discipline if you seriously intend to achieve any worthwhile goals in life.

It's not always going to be easy, and it's not always going to be fun. However, **it will hurt you more in the**

long run if you do not discipline yourself to do the right thing.

Every act you perform is motivated either by your desire to avoid pain or to gain pleasure. More often than not, your need to avoid pain is a stronger stimulus for your actions than your desire for pleasure, particularly if the pleasure is long-term.

For example, you want to earn a higher income in your current job or you want to start a new business. You realise that you will need to spend some extra time studying to improve your skills in order to achieve that goal.

But you would rather spend your spare time catching up on the soaps on TV (a pleasurable act for you – no stress involved). The idea of sacrificing TV time for study seems 'painful' compared with the alternative. So you decide to watch TV as usual instead.

Time comes for promotion and you get passed over (because you haven't shown any sign of progress in your work). You begin to complain about how unfair life is, since you've been in that company for the past decade. You then regret not making the effort to improve your chances at work.

Another example is the smoker who continues to smoke even though he is aware of the deadly consequences of the habit. The (perceived) pain he associates with not smoking keeps him addicted to it. He figures it is more painful to stop smoking than it is to deal with his underlying reason for wanting to smoke. Because the health dangers associated with smoking develop gradually, he does not feel the (very real) pain of smoking-related illness until it is too late. Then, on his death bed, he is filled with regret about the things he did, did not do or should have done.

Regret is painful. But discipline can be 'painful' too, depending on how you look at it. However, the pain of regret is longer lasting and more severe, whereas the 'pain' of discipline is short-lived and leads to enormous pleasure (self-respect, satisfaction, higher income, etc) in the end. In other words, regret hurts more than discipline does.

Any form of discipline 'hurts', but it's only for a while. The regret you feel when you do not get the things you want in life as a result of your lack of self-discipline hurts more and doesn't lead to any positive results (unless it pushes you to go discipline yourself).

Here is an illustration from real-life that will hopefully drive the point home.

When I first started to practise medicine, I came across many patients suffering from Type II Diabetes Mellitus. Now this condition is potentially devastating yet 100% controllable by healthy lifestyle practices.

Yet I had many patients who, as a result of lack of self-discipline, (they continued to smoke, eat unhealthy foods, refused to exercise etc), ended up blind, with kidney failure, leg ulcers needing amputation and other horrible complications. Totally unnecessary.

None of these complications had to happen to those patients. However because they considered it 'painful' or 'difficult' to control their lifestyle habits, they ended up shortening their lifespan and making their existing lives of the poorest quality. Trust me, those of them that needed amputations literally felt the pain of regret ('if only I had watched my diet', 'if only I had started exercising when the doctor first told me to', 'if only I had stopped smoking', 'if only...' - none of which could bring back the legs they had lost).

You see, you have to make a choice if you are to succeed: discipline now or regret later. Next time you feel like procrastinating or not doing something you know you should, ask yourself which will hurt you more - the end result of doing it or the end result of not doing it.

Choose which 'pain' you would rather bear because you will bear some 'pain' on your way. That's just the way life is. You can either choose the relative 'pain' of discipline (which is short-lived and has great rewards for you at the end) or the definite and absolute 'pain' of regret which is long-lasting and can sometimes be devastating as some things are irreversible.

Having said this though, there are ways to make discipline less 'painful'. That will be dealt with in a future publication. Main thing is for you to make a conscious choice today that you would rather 'suffer' now briefly for a greater reward the rest of your life, than 'enjoy' briefly and have a lifetime of regret (which is real suffering).

The following exercise is designed to help you practise self-discipline until it becomes a habit. Do not just read it. Get your pen and paper and do it. Success is the result of action, not wishing or just reading.

EXERCISE

- Name two things you could do today which, if you did them every day, would make a big difference in your life.

- What keeps you from doing each one? What thoughts prevent you from taking action?

- How would you feel if, at the end of your life, you had not accomplished the results you would otherwise have done from each action?

- Start doing one or both actions today. Decide to commit to doing this no matter what. Engage the power of your will power and self discipline to make this happen.

NOTES

"I hated every minute of training, but I said, 'Don't quit. Suffer now and live the rest of your life as a champion."
Muhammad Ali

DAY 14
CURE THE WORRY HABIT

"I believe God is managing affairs and that He doesn't need any advice from me. With God in charge, I believe everything will work out for the best in the end. So what is there to worry about?"
Henry Ford

Do you ever find yourself struggling to achieve something or to become something or to do something, yet never seem to get the results you desire?

Ever catch yourself worrying about the outcome of an interview or presentation or conversation? You really want things to turn out well but you find yourself worrying that they may not?

If you have, then I have news for you.

The very act of worrying repels the thing you want from coming to you.

You've probably heard about the so called 'Law of Attraction'. It's called 'Attraction' because the things you want get drawn (or attracted) to you with minimal effort on your part when you meet the right conditions.

One of the conditions you need to meet in order to attract the things you want is to **let go** of your worries and struggling attitude.

When you know what you want and you know what to do in order to get it, then do it and leave it at that. Don't waste precious time and energy agonising over how things will turn out.

Worrying sends out a subconscious message that 'I don't have what I want' or 'I lack what I want' and in doing so, you attract more of the lack you're worried about.

Think of a farmer. He plants his seeds at the right season. His 'goal' or desired outcome is to have a bountiful harvest come harvest time. He knows he has to take care of the crops as they grow, nourish them with manure, water them, get rid of weeds and so on. So he gets on with it and does what he knows he needs to do.

What if he spent time worrying about what sort of harvest he'd get. What if, every morning he ran out to his farm to see if his harvest has come. You'd think he was nuts, right?

What does he do instead, our farmer? He gets on with his life, that's what. He **fully believes** that harvest time will come, and because he's **taking the right steps** (appropriate action) to ensure a good harvest, he doesn't waste time worrying about what sort of crops he'll reap.

Worrying is futile. It doesn't solve anything. Worst of all, it actually repels the very thing you want to attract.

As someone has said, **"Worry is like a rocking chair, it will give you something to do, but it won't get you anywhere".**

These principles are beautiful and powerful because they apply to anybody who chooses to abide by them.

Do not worry about anything. Worrying does not solve problems. Rather, it prevents you from seeking and finding solutions to the problems. Fear, agitation and anxiety do not move you towards your goals. They paralyse you and repel your desired outcome instead. Appropriate action always brings you closer to what you want though. As does gratitude for what you do have right now.

So from now onwards, any time you are tempted to be afraid or to worry about whether you will get what you want, STOP! Instead, give thanks for something good in your life right now, then DO SOMETHING that will move you towards the outcome you desire, then get on with your life.

And if you sometimes worry about what people think of you, which is a colossal waste of time, here is a quote for you to remember:

> "We would worry less about what others think of us if we realised how seldom they do."
> Ethel Barrett

The opinions of others about you have no bearing on your life whatsoever, unless you give them that power. So don't even go there.

Love and respect yourself and don't lose any sleep over if anyone else does.

EXERCISE

How To Ditch The Worry Habit

- What bugs you?

- What do you worry about?

- From this day on, practise giving yourself this command: "I now let go of my concern about......." (fill in the blank with whatever issue/s cause you to worry). You could also say "I now release myself from worry" or "I am now free from worry" - practise the command that sounds and feels most comfortable to you.

'Ditch The Worry Habit' on steroids

- If you are prone to worrying, wear a rubber band around your wrist. Any time you catch yourself worrying, snap the rubber band around your wrist and speak your chosen 'command phrase' to yourself.

- Basically in today's exercise, you're replacing one habit (the bad habit of worrying) with another habit (a good one).

- Practise this until you don't need to wear your ubber band to remember to stop worrying.

IT's simple but powerful and effective. As Jim Rohn would say, it's easy to do and easy not to do.

NOTES

*"What's the use of worrying? It never was worth while,
so pack up your troubles in your old
kit-bag, and smile, smile, smile."
George Asaf*

DAY 15
SYSTEMS ARE THE KEY TO YOUR SUCCESS

"Systems put your success on autopilot"
Dr Nkem Ezeilo

You've probably heard the saying 'Success leaves clues'. It may be a cliché, but it's true. One of the 'clues' that successful people leave is that they have a system that leads them to success.

Think about any highly successful person you know. You will find that they didn't just stumble upon their great achievements. They knew what they wanted to achieve, then followed a proven system to help them get there.

You have an 'operating system' for your life right now, whether or not you're aware of it. Of course, the ideal thing is for you not only to be aware of it, but to be the author and controller of your own system. That way, when things don't go according to plan, you know where the problem is and you can fix it and move on.

You have a system of thinking and doing things right now. The way your life is currently is the result of the operating system you have used up until now.
How do you operate?

If your life seems chaotic and directionless, it means you have a system of chaos. Like it or not, you live by some system or other.

If you have been unaware of this, now is the time to wake up and question the way things are. Are you happy with the way things are in your life right now? Would you rather be doing something else? Would you like to enjoy perfect health and have lots of energy regardless of how busy your schedule is? Would you like to earn more money than you are doing at the moment? Want to stop smoking?

What do you want? You can achieve all the above and more, but you need to have a system in place to help you get there. Nature is organised and orderly. You must become organised in order to get what you want. A system helps you stay organised.

For you to succeed in any venture you undertake, get clear on the outcome you desire. Then come up with a plan or system that will lead you to your desired outcome.

Once you have a system in place, **be persistent.** Realise that your results may not happen instantly. Do not get discouraged about the rate at which things are going. Rest assured that **'in all labour there is profit'.** In good time your system will pay off.

Having a system gives you more time to do things you want to do. It makes you confident and keeps you on top of things - no more feeling scattered and disorganised. Perhaps this acronym for the word 'systems' will give you a better understanding:

Save
Yourself
Substantial
Time
Energy
Money and
Stress

Of course your system has to be the right one for the result you hope to achieve. Always be flexible and open enough to see when something isn't working so you can change it.

When you know what you want to accomplish, you can even develop inter-related systems, which work in synchrony to help you do many things at the same time. Let me illustrate by sharing a bit of my system with you:

My health goal is to keep my body weight at a certain level for optimal health (you don't need to know my weight details…). My spiritual goal is to be thoroughly familiar with the Laws of the Universe and apply these consciously daily. My marketing goal is to add at least 100 new subscribers each day to my mailing list. My mental/intellectual goal is to be on top of things in my career and personal development (I've summarised the goals to save space).

So when I wake up, I do what I call 'the 3 Ws': Worship, Work-out and Write (and submit articles). During my work-out I listen to self-improvement tapes for at least 30 minutes. Without going into further detail, you can see how following this simple system consistently leads to the results I desire in each of those areas. There's more of course, but you get the picture.

There's just no other possible outcome: nature operates on the premise of cause and effect. If I work out regularly and eat right for instance, the only possible result is that I stay healthy and fit provided all other things (known as Ten Pillars of Health, particularly the Mindset Pillar) are on point. But notice how each 'W' helps me accomplish a different goal. So just doing 'the 3 Ws' daily brings me closer to my desired outcome in three different areas of my life. That's synchrony. That's a working system.

The key thing is to **find out what works for you**, make it fun and simple, and stick to it. And reward yourself every step of the way, any time you successfully accomplish any part of your system. That will help you stay motivated even when you don't yet see results (some things take a while to show up).

As with every new habit, you may find it difficult to follow your new system but it's well worth every effort to persist. After all, your old/current system isn't working (if it is, and you're happy with the way things are, then keep it up - 'if it ain't broke, don't fix it').

Find out what your system is. It is your current way of doing things. Your current way of operating. If you seek it, you will find it. Adjust it so that it steers you in the direction of the outcomes you desire for your life. Determine what is your ideal outcome in each area of your life. Then **create a personal system** that will lead you to success in each area.

If you don't have a clue about what sort of system to use, seek out people who have succeeded in each area. Find out what they have done. Personalise their system to reflect your values and needs. Then work your new system. Persist until you succeed because if you stick to your system consistently, you WILL get the results you desire.

EXERCISE

- Choose one of your goals for this exercise: which of your goals do you first wish to create a system for reaching?

- What steps are involved in accomplishing this goal?

- Which of those steps involve activities that recur? Write them down.

- Write out a possible system for achieving this goal.

- Test and modify it until you have a fluent system that works for you.

NOTES

"Once you have a clear picture of your priorities- that is values, goals, and high leverage activities- organize around them."
Stephen Covey

DAY 16
AFFIRMATIONS – HOW TO MAKE THEM WORK FOR YOU

"I figured that if I said it enough, I would convince the world that I really was the greatest."
Muhammad Ali

You have probably heard about affirmations so many times. All the 'gurus' claim to use them, and tell you how effective they are.

You may even have given them a shot, the best way you know how, yet everything stays the same in your life. So you've concluded that affirmations don't work. You've decided that they're just hype. Feel-good stuff that doesn't make any difference whatsoever.

If that describes you or someone you know, then read this chapter very carefully, because the wrong conception could be preventing you from benefiting from this powerful, free and effective tool.

Affirmations do work, but **only** when you do them right. Yes, you should state them positively. You should state them in the present. You should really want what you're affirming and all that. But there is usually one vital ingredient missing in the picture when people talk to me about their affirmations.

What's that ingredient? **Belief. Faith.** You say one thing with your mouth, but in your heart you do not believe what you are saying.

Your affirmation is not believable to you where it matters most - in your subconscious mind. This cancels out your efforts and make your affirmations ineffective.

Let's illustrate this with an example.

You want to manage your time better. So you write down an affirmation 'I am efficient in my use of time'. You say it however many times you've been told to say it each day. Each time you say it, a voice inside you goes, 'yeah right, says who?'. Throughout the day you do things you know you shouldn't do (time-wasting activities) and come night-time, you faithfully affirm once again: 'I am efficient in my use of time'.

Weeks and then months go by and you don't notice any difference.

Sound familiar?

Your affirmations won't work if you do not believe that what you say happens. Now if you've been reading this book for any length of time, you'll remember that **believing something implies <u>acting</u> in a way that's**

congruent to your beliefs. If you say you
believe something, yet behave in a way that
contradicts what you claim to believe, then the truth is
you don't believe that thing.

So in our example above, if you want to make your
affirmation believable and thus effective, back it up
with appropriate actions. Action speaks louder than
words. Well, the right action speaks louder than even
those inner words that we hear inside of us that try to
put us down and keep us from achieving the results
we desire.

To make your affirmation work (using the example
above), map out a plan of action to help you
manage your time better. Decide to do first things first.
Eliminate unnecessary activities from your daily routine.
Make a plan, then work your plan. That way, when
you say 'I am efficient in my use of time', it will be
easier for you to believe it.

Another way to make your affirmations effective by
making them believable to you, is to **state them in a progressive way.** Emile Coué, the great psychiatrist,
put it best. He got his clients to say 'everyday and in
everyway, by the grace of God, I am getting better
and better'. He had them say it daily. Notice that they
were saying they were improving daily, not that they
were already there.

This progressive method of affirming things makes it easier for you to believe what you are saying. Think about it. If, when you look in the mirror, you see an overweight body, then you affirm: 'I am slim, toned and fit'. How do you feel saying that? Like a fraud, right? You'd feel like you have just lied, because you have, in fact, lied. But if you say (paraphrasing Coué) 'Everyday and in everyway, by the grace of God, I am getting fitter and slimmer', **then promptly back it up with appropriate action** (exercise, eat healthy food, take quality supplements, eliminate stress etc) – you would believe your affirmations, wouldn't you? They would then become more effective for you.

Remember, faith in what you're saying makes affirmations work. It not only motivates you to continue acting in a way that brings your goals to pass. It also attracts things into your life which pull you towards your goals.

> Faith makes affirmations work.

One more way to help you believe in your affirmations is by **believing in something bigger than yourself.** Believe that God wants to help you be, do and have all that is best for you. That way you know you are not alone. Most of the great, highly successful people that ever lived testify to the amazing power of this sort of faith.

When you believe inspired words such as the ones in the Bible or other similar literature, then it makes it easy for you to make affirmations in the present. After all (you believe), God said it so it must be true.

For example, there's a verse in the Bible that says **'If you believe in your heart that the things you say shall come to pass, then they shall be done for you'** (paraphrasing Mark 11: 23). Now if those words were said by some wino on the street, you would not believe him because he has no credibility. As a result, they would not be effective affirmations for you.

But when you realise who said them, and make affirmations based on them, based on your faith or belief in the integrity of the source of those words (which is a choice you make, remember), your affirmations WILL bring about the results you desire. I say this from personal experience. I have personally used that verse to 'dictate' events in my life before they've occurred.

Always remember that whenever I talk about faith and believing, it must be backed with appropriate action in order to be effective.

Never think for one second that all you have to do is think positive and affirm and you'll get what you want.

Affirmations and positive thoughts are simply tools that put you in the right frame of mind to take the right action, and to persist in it until you get your desired results.

Back your faith with action if you want to succeed.

"Faith without works is dead"
The Bible

In summary, let us review the ways you can begin TODAY to make your affirmations powerful and effective. Let's summarise the ways to make your affirmations believable.

- Map out a **plan of action that supports your affirmation** then work your plan.

- State your affirmation in a **progressive** way, Coué-style.

- **Believe** that God is willing to help you be, do, have the best things in life. Then go through the Bible or other inspired writings, looking for quotes you can personalise and use as your affirmations. Write them down and read through them daily. Out loud if possible.

These things work, but you have got to do them right.

EXERCISE

Affirmations are sentences that describe a desired goal. They work by empowering you to control your thoughts (as you know, you are what you think.).

Practise with one of your goals – turn it into an affirmation, using the following principles:

- To make affirmations work for you,

- They must be believable. This will help you achieve your goals faster. Having said that, if you continue to repeat your affirmations, you will eventually start to believe the things you are saying. Still, isn't it better to start the process with a basic level of faith? I've found it to help.

- State them in the present tense, or in the progressive form (like Coué).

- Use positive wording. If for example your goal is to pass an exam, don't affirm 'I won't fail this exam'. Instead, say 'I will pass this exam'.

- They should be personal to you.

- They should arouse some emotion in you. This is one place where it helps if you believe in what you're saying. If you believe you'll get what you're affirming, then the mere act of affirming it will make you feel good, joyous, positive. Try it and see.

- GAP and write down your affirmations.

- Say them out loud or read them at least twice each day – at least once when you wake up, and once just before you go to bed at night. Repetition, and persistence in doing so, WILL bring you the results you want.

- Back your affirmations with appropriate action. You can't affirm your way to a good job or better health unless you are taking the right steps to lead you there.

NOTES

"Affirmation without discipline is the beginning of delusion."
Jim Rohn

DAY 17
LISTENING TO YOUR INNER VOICE

> "What you hear repeatedly you will eventually believe."
> Mike Murdock

Do you suffer from low self-esteem? Do you sometimes feel like your life is not worth living? Perhaps you feel you will never rise above your current status in life. Ever stopped to analyse the thoughts behind those feelings at the time?

If you did, you would notice that the times you feel negative about yourself, you are thinking pretty bad thoughts about yourself. Put another way, you are listening to the wrong voice within.

We all have two 'voices' speaking to us most of the time. These voices are actually just thoughts that occupy our minds. They are contradictory in nature: one line of thought (voice) is positive and constructive. The trouble is, a lot of the time you ignore what this good voice says – probably because it can be quiet and unforceful.

This is the voice that, for example, will give you good ideas and encourage you to try them. When you do act on these good ideas, you become very successful at them. This same quiet voice tells you that you can do it (or as I teach in my Confidence Course for Women, it tells you that really, 'you're all that and a bag of kale crisps!'). It tells you the truth about yourself, if you would dare to believe it. It reminds you of the good things you've accomplished, the good things others have said about you.

The second voice is negative and destructive. It rushes to put you down at the first hint of progress in any area of your life. It's that inner 'demon' or 'gremlin' as some call it, and we all have one. I call it 'your personal saboteur'. It tells you you're no good, who do you think you are, you're a failure, and so many other things designed to spoil your plans and keep you under. It reminds you of the mistakes you've made and the negative things people have said about you. It tries to make you doubt yourself and your abilities (and it succeeds if you let it).

The problem with this is that more often than not, you believe the thoughts are true. Here's something for you to think about:

The fact that you hold a thought in your mind does not make that thought true.

It's up to you to **choose which thoughts you will hold true**. If you want to achieve any worthwhile objective, then reject thoughts that prevent you from achieving it. If you don't, these thoughts will become beliefs - so-called **limiting beliefs** because they limit you from attempting and achieving things you otherwise would.

Rather, decide to listen to that other voice inside you, the quiet one that encourages you to 'go for it', 'you can do it'. Agree with that voice that whispers good things about you. These thoughts empower you to achieve success when you hold them in your mind consistently. Turn up the volume of your 'inner cheerleader' (also known as your 'inner motivator') and turn down the volume of your 'inner saboteur'.

> *"If you don't change your beliefs, your life will be like this forever.*
> *Is that good news?"*
> Dr. Robert Anthony

Remember that if you think a certain thought long enough, you start to believe it's true. And what you believe determines your behaviour. Your behaviour determines the results you get in life.

Choose today who you are going to listen to. Which of your inner voices will have the upper hand? What are you going to believe about yourself? About others? About the world?

Once you have a sound belief in yourself and your abilities, it won't matter what others think or say. You will be self-assured and won't need others' approval in order to feel good about yourself.

It pays to listen to the right voices. Have you watched the movie 'A Beautiful Mind'? That film perfectly illustrates the concept of 'voices'. As long as Russell Crowe's character listened to the 'crazy voices' in his head, he acted abnormally. At the end of the movie, he had mastered his thoughts such that, even though the crazy voices never left, they now had no effect on him whatsoever. He then went on to win a Nobel prize.

You see, your 'inner saboteur' will always be there. You might well accept that fact and decide to stop listening to it.

The following exercise shows you how to eliminate limiting beliefs (and thus conquer your 'inner gremlin') once and for all. It will only work if you actually do the exercise.

EXERCISE

- Time to whip out that old rubber band again.

- The trick with your inner saboteur is not to deny its existence, but rather to acknowledge it and then choose to move on with other activities.

- In other words, you're taking your attention away from it by focusing it elsewhere, on a more productive, worthwhile task.

- So put on your rubber band around your wrist.

- Any time you catch yourself listening to your inner gremlin, snap the rubber band real hard and change what you're doing at once. You could also loudly speak out the opposite of what that voice is saying.

- Keep a progress diary to track how you're doing.

- You will notice that many of these exercises employ the same theme. The reason for this is simple: mental reprogramming is not an overnight job. It's taken you years of bad programming to land you where you are right now.

- This programming or conditioning needs to be overwritten with more powerful, empowering stuff. That's what these daily exercises are designed to do for you if you work through them.

NOTES

"Don't let the noise of others' opinions drown out your own inner voice."
Steve Jobs

DAY 18
DECLUTTER YOUR LIFE

*"Small ills are the fountains of most of our groans.
Men trip not on mountains, they stumble on stones."*
Chinese Proverb

Have you ever noticed how light you feel after doing a thorough cleaning job? Sometimes just clearing the top of your desk leaves you feeling refreshed and raring to go. Ever wondered why?

It's an interesting phenomenon. What happens is that the clearing process creates a 'vacuum' (and we know that nature abhors a vacuum). The 'vacuum' in turn stimulates a surge of 'oomph' or creative energy, which is designed to get you to fill it up.

Now the ball is in your court. You can fill up that vacuum by doing worthless stuff (which will leave you feeling cluttered, drained and frustrated again), or you can fill it up by doing worthwhile stuff (which will maintain your 'oomph').

Another way to apply this principle is this. If you want to attract the things you desire into your life, first make room for them by eliminating the things you don't want from your life. When you have 'cleared' those unwanted things (including unproductive relationships) from your life, you will feel renewed and refreshed.

You will have a burst of positive energy just waiting for you to apply to something good.

To attract the things you want into your life, use your newly-found positive energy to do things which will bring about the results you desire. An amazing thing happens when you do this.

Things, people and circumstances come your way, which help you get closer to your goals. You begin to notice a lot of 'coincidences' (coincidence? I think not!), all of which seem designed to pull you and your desires together.

This works because you are correctly applying a universal principle.

Try it today. Begin with outward de-cluttering - tidy up your office desk, your room, your kitchen, whichever part of your environment that needs cleaning up. Do a thorough job, and be brutal with your junk. Get rid of stuff you don't need. Stuff you haven't used in a year. Delete emails you won't read.

Practise on the outer stuff, and with the 'oomph' you get by doing that, get to work on the inner stuff (see below). You will be much happier and fulfilled when you do. Or you could work on both. Just don't let yourself become overwhelmed by everything you have to do. Do it in baby steps.

Notice that overcoming procrastination is a perfect example of getting rid of things you're putting up with. In this case you would be getting rid of a dangerous habit. So if you've got a problem with procrastination, read the next chapter.

Another term for the phrase 'putting up with something' is **toleration.** A toleration is something (or someone) that you would be better off without. Tolerations sap your life of fun and enthusiasm. They drain you and make your life a drag. Do everything you can to eliminate tolerations from your life.

De-clutter your life today and become a **'toleration-free zone.'**

The following exercise will show you how.

Tolerate nothing

EXERCISE

- De-cluttering your life becomes easy when you first apply it to physical things.

- Look around your environment: your home/office, wherever you spend a lot of time.

- Go through the rooms and pick out things you have no need of.

- Be brutal about it. Don't let sentiment keep you stuck in a rut – if you haven't used it in a year, get rid of it, whatever 'it' is. This is also a way of practising letting go.

- There are various ways of disposing of the things you're getting rid of – give them to charity, sell them on ebay, give them to friends or simply throw them away.

- Outward clutter is a reflection of inner clutter. If your home or environment is cluttered, it is evidence that your mind is cluttered as well.

- What's wrong with a cluttered mind, I hear you ask?

- A cluttered mind repels everything good. Rather it attracts more of the same. It attracts negative energy, which leaves you feeling drained and lethargic all the time.

- So get on with it today. Don't get overwhelmed by the task ahead of you though; baby steps are the key to your success. Devote 10-15 minutes each day to de-cluttering your home. Write in your success journal how you feel at the end of it all.

- Starting now.

NOTES

*"Nothing is as fatiguing as the continued hanging on of
an uncompleted task."*
William James

DAY 19
HOW TO CONQUER PROCRASTINATION

"Procrastination is opportunity's assassin."
Victor Kiam

Procrastination – putting off things – is a habit that is easy to cultivate. The trouble is, it's a bad (and sometimes dangerous) habit. Like all bad habits, it doesn't take much effort to form. That's why it's easy to fall into the trap.

There are several ways in which procrastination sabotages your efforts. I have listed a few below:

- **It wastes your time:** if there's something you're supposed to do and you postpone doing it, you know you'll have to do it eventually. If you don't do it when you're supposed to, you'll end up doing it when you should be doing something else.

- **It lowers your self-esteem:** you feel you have failed if by the end of the day you have not done what you should have. This eats at your self esteem and your image of yourself is not a good one.

- **It keeps you from reaching your goals.**

- **It gives you a false sense of comfort:** you deceive yourself when you think 'I'll do it later'. You never know what might come up later, making it impossible to do the task.

- **It is a sign of laziness.** Chances are, if you're lazy in one aspect of your life, you're lazy in other aspects as well. Scary thought.

- **It keeps things piling up.** This makes you feel overwhelmed when you finally get round to doing them. A vicious cycle then develops because you are put off by how much you now have to do.

- Procrastination **keeps you stuck.** It prevents you from progressing in life.

- **You cannot concentrate** on doing other tasks until you've completed the one at hand. You feel like there's 'unfinished business', which there is.

Since you're not totally focused on any given task (because other undone tasks are on your mind), you do a shoddy job. This sets up another vicious cycle because you have to come back and correct the mistakes you've made. What a waste of time.

There are many more disadvantages of procrastinating but I hope the few I've listed above have helped you realise it's time to break the habit.

If they have, that's good.

I have put together my top five tips for overcoming procrastination. These work a treat.

Read them, put them into practice and see the results for yourself.

Top Five Tips For Overcoming Procrastination

1. **Do your least favourite tasks first.**
   Get them over and done with, and then subsequent tasks will seem more enjoyable.

2. **Decide to 'Do It Now'!**
   Let that be your mantra, then go ahead and DO IT NOW.

3. **Think of 5 benefits of doing it now.**
   For instance:

   - You get more time to do other things.

   - You get an increased sense of accomplishment, which leads to greater self-esteem. You feel very good about yourself.

   - You don't feel stuck because you're getting things done: you feel free to move onto other tasks.

   - You can concentrate on other tasks, so you do them better.

- You reach your goals faster.

4. **Keep a record of your progress.**
   This will motivate and encourage you to continue the habit of doing things now.

5. **Break down each task** into smaller, easily manageable chunks. Then apply points 1 to 4 above to each chunk.

Follow the above tips and you will begin to conquer the evil that is procrastination.

Persevere in doing them and you will overcome it for good.

One last thing: start doing them NOW!

EXERCISE

- Name one activity or task you've been putting off.

- Remind yourself what's important about that task: why should you do it? What will it cost you not to do it now?

- What stops you from doing it now?

- What steps (if any) do you need to take in order to do it?

- Go ahead and take the first step towards that task now.

NOTES

"Procrastination is the bad habit of putting of until the day after tomorrow what should have been done the day before yesterday".
Napoleon Hill

DAY 20
DO IT NOW

"You may delay, but time will not."
Benjamin Franklin

The concept of 'doing it now', introduced in the previous chapter, is so crucial to your success that it deserves a separate chapter.

One difference between the 'haves' and the 'have nots', or the 'successful' and the 'unsuccessful' people of our world, is in what they have or have not **done.**

Successful women are women of action. They act on ideas, instead of sitting and dreaming or just talking about them.

Remember, every achievement or success story started as an idea in someone's mind. Everyone has ideas, some of them brilliant ones even, but **not everyone acts on their ideas**. Did you ever have an idea that you did not act on? Then when someone else got a similar idea and acted on it, with good results? Did you start to whinge, saying that you thought of it first?

Like that makes any difference!

I'm all for having ideas and I believe in positive thinking, affirmations and the other success principles more than anything, but in my opinion, they're all worthless until you back them up with ACTION (Appropriate Action – see day 11).

If that (the vital importance of TAKING ACTION) is the only thing you take away from reading this book then it would have been worth my while writing it.

Many people remain poor because they were too scared to act on a money-making idea they had. Perhaps that has happened to you or someone you know. You've had this great idea, but because you're concerned about what others will think of you when you act on it, you do nothing about it. Guess who loses out in the end.

The fact is, the sooner you act on your ideas, the sooner you know for sure which ones work and which ones don't. And the sooner you can keep on trying out different ideas until you get the results you want.

Always remember this: if you want to do something, the very desire to do it is an indication that you CAN do it.

Read that statement again. I like the way it's put in the Bible: **the One who gives you the desire to do something has also given you the ability to do it well** (my paraphrase).

So be bold. Learn that new instrument. Start that business. Ask that guy or girl out on a date. Take that course or get that degree. Write that story or novel. Hire that life coach!

Whatever you want to do, know that you can do it and do it now.

Don't worry about what anyone else will think. It's your life after all, and trying out new things is part of what makes life exciting and interesting. Sure you'll make mistakes along the way but it's all part of the learning experience.

EXERCISE

- What one thing have you wanted to do but been too afraid to even try?

- What idea do you have which, if you could pull it off, could lead to your breakthrough?

- What step could you take today, now, in the direction of that idea?

- Take that step NOW! After that, take the next step.

- Don't be afraid to make mistakes – if babies were afraid of making mistakes they'd never learn how to walk.

NOTES

*"Seize this very minute! Boldness has genius, power, and magic in it.
Only engage, and then the mind grows heated.
Begin, and then the work will be completed."
John Anster*

DAY 21
HOW DO YOU SEE THINGS?

"To different minds, the same world is a hell, and a heaven."
Ralph Waldo Emerson

There's something interesting about life as we know it. Our attitudes determine our responses to various events or stimuli. Our responses in turn determine our experience of the events or stimuli.

The events themselves remain the same; they are neither good nor bad. However the way we experience events varies, **depending on our interpretation** of what is happening.

Here is an illustration: SD recently joined a firm as an associate. She seemed aloof most of the time, and DT, a co-worker, concluded that SD was being snobbish. She then decided to make things difficult for SD ('that'll teach her to ignore me when I greet her. Who does she think she is anyway?').

DT's plan was to start a nasty rumour about SD during lunch break. Come lunch break, (SD was by herself in the office as usual) DT brought up the topic of SD with the girls. "Guess what I heard about SD:...", she said, and then rattled off a trail of made-up stories, all designed to make SD look bad.

MG, one of the girls in the group, spoke up: "That can't be true, DT. I've known SD for a while now and that's not her way of doing things. The poor thing, do you know she recently lost her fiancé in a car accident? I can't imagine the pain she's going through now."

Guess how DT felt to learn that SD's 'snobbish behaviour' wasn't intentional, but was really her way of dealing with her grief.

DT felt awful about how wrong she had read the SD situation. She then decided to amend things as soon as possible. Before lunch break was over, she excused herself and went to find SD. She struck up a conversation with SD, hoping to make friends with her. To her pleasant surprise, DT found SD to be a really nice person who just still hadn't gotten over the loss of her loved one. They eventually became fast friends, and with DT's help, SD was able to heal quickly and return to her normal, bubbly self.

Notice that the only thing that had changed in the whole picture was DT's interpretation of SD's behaviour. DT began to see SD in a different light once she had her facts straight. This changed her behaviour towards SD as a result.

Very often we assume things or interpret things **based on our past experiences, thoughts and expectations.** Much of the time, our assumptions are not based on facts. Consequently, they may turn out to be wrong.

To make things worse, we then say things or do things based on our false interpretations of events.

This sort of thing hurts several people, including the person making the false assumption. It also destroys interpersonal relationships.

One sure-fire way to avoid reading the wrong meaning into things is by seeking out the facts. Ask questions of the right people. Do not assume that because things look a certain way (to you) then that's the way things are.

In the context of a relationship, this means you should communicate with the person in question and find out things for yourself.

It's a healthy way to deal with things, and you get to sleep better at night for it, knowing things for sure, instead of just guessing.

Another sure-fire way is to assume that the other person means well (until they prove otherwise). Seek to understand where they're coming from, seek to understand the reason for their behaviour if it doesn't match the 'meaning well' premise. Don't jump to conclusions without this full understanding. It may surprise you to learn that people are generally all right, and things aren't as bad as they look.

Change the way you see things, and the things you see will change.

Really, **'there's nothing good or bad, only thinking makes it so'.** (Shakespeare)

EXERCISE

Something to think about:

- You can't read anyone's mind so don't assume anything when relating to people. Think of the times when you've treated someone one way based on an assumption you had about them, only to wish you'd known all the facts before treating them that way.

- How will you put this principle into practice today? There are certain things you can't change in this life, but one thing you can change is the way you see things, your perception, your interpretation of things.

- How can you interpret things in ways that empower you?

- When someone says something about you, rather than think they had ulterior motives when saying it, how could you interpret this such that your interpretation leaves you feeling empowered?

- From today, choose to 'read' people and circumstances in ways that empower you - that is, make you feel good about yourself and and them, and leave you in such a resourceful state that you can achieve any task you set for yourself.

NOTES

"Change the way you look at things and the things you look at change."
Wayne W. Dyer

DAY 22
GET A MENTAL WORK-OUT

"Questions focus our thinking. Ask empowering questions like: What's good about this? What's not perfect about it yet? What am I going to do next time? How can I do this and have fun doing it?"
Charles Connolly

Just as your body needs a regular work-out to stay fit, functional and healthy, your mind needs one too, for the same reason.

Questions are a great way of exercising your mind and giving it a work-out.

Whenever you face a dilemma that seems unsolvable, give yourself a mental work-out by asking yourself the right questions.

The right questions make you think of a solution to the problem. They get your mind working (even while you sleep) until you come up with the right answer to your question.

For instance, if you're stuck in a day job but you'd rather be your own boss and have a flexible, fulfilled life, don't ask 'Why do I lead such a drab existence?' or some such question. If you do, your mind will start working hard to find out just why your life is drab.

Imagine how depressed you'll feel when that's all you think about.

Instead ask yourself 'How can I get out of this situation? How can I create the lifestyle I want? What can I do today to make my life better?'. This second line of questioning will immediately get your mind working to find the right answer to that question. You will feel upbeat and hopeful. Better still, you will begin to have all sorts of ideas to try out. One of those ideas will be the one you're looking for.

Whenever I want to create an extra source of income in a short time, I ask myself 'What can I do to earn £.... in (so many) days?' I always specify the exact amount I need and the exact time frame I need it in. Without fail, the answer comes to me. Not always instantly, but definitely eventually. It comes in form of ideas that had not occurred to me before.

If you want to make your life more enjoyable, ask 'What can I do to make my life more fun-filled?' or something similar. Next time you see something you would like to buy, and the 'I can't afford it' thought creeps up, immediately change it to a question 'How can I raise the cash to enable me to buy this thing?'

After you ask these questions, pay attention to the thoughts that occur to you. Begin to act on the ones that appeal to you. Do not wait for conditions to be perfect before you act. Action has the power to make things happen.

So begin today to monitor the questions you ask yourself.

You will be surprised what a little regular mental workout can do for you.

Go ahead and do it. When you think of the possible results you can have, don't you feel excited? Just ask yourself how to make it happen, and get to work with the ideas you come up with.

Enjoy your mental workout!

"It's not the answer that enlightens, but the question."
Decouvertes

EXERCISE

- Refer again to your goals sheet.

- Pick one of your goals. What questions could you ask yourself about it, whose answers would bring you closer to accomplishing the goal?

- Brainstorm as many as you can think of and write them down.

- Any time you need to focus or concentrate on a (goal-related) task, ask yourself questions about it. Asking questions causes your brain to focus on seeking the solution to the question.

NOTES

"If you do not ask the right questions, you do not get the right answers. A question asked in the right way often points to its own answer. Asking questions is the A-B-C of diagnosis. Only the inquiring mind solves problems."
Edward Hodnett

DAY 23
HOW TO BE SELFISH TO SUCCEED

"Drop the idea that you are Atlas carrying the world on your shoulders. The world would go on even without you. Don't take yourself so seriously."
Norman Vincent Peale

Today, I will show you why you need to be a selfish person and how to become one!

Before you think I've gone nuts, let me explain what I mean. When I say 'selfish' in this article, I don't mean self-serving or selfish to the detriment or exclusion of others.

What I'm referring to here is something noble. It means 'take extreme care of yourself first'. It refers to loving yourself in order to make you able to love your neighbour.

Guess what your most valuable asset on this planet is? You are!

Think about it: you are the only version of you in existence. You are the only one with your unique combination of talents, abilities, faults and all.

In your relationships, **you** are a special part of the equation.

If you want to earn an income, **you** have to make it happen.
If you want to be there for your family, **you** have to be there.
Life throws so many things at you and you need to be in good shape if you're to handle them properly.

Even the Bible says to **'love your neighbour as you love yourself'**. That clearly implies that you should love yourself first, or else how can you love someone else?

Remember the safety instructions you receive when you board an airplane? They tell you to sort out yourself first (put on your oxygen mask and so on) before you sort out your own children.

What does that tell you?

In plain terms, you need to be in 'good working condition' before you can be of any use to yourself or anyone else.

If you are sick and/or stressed out all the time, your performance at work and home is affected. That usually sets up a vicious cycle where you may end up losing your job or your loved ones in the worst case scenario.

All because you have not taken care of or nurtured yourself.

You have a spirit, a soul and a body. Begin today to take care of each of those aspects of your life. Do it in a balanced way, as none is more important than the other.

10 Tips to help you become 'selfish' (in a good way)

- Take regular exercise (it improves quality and length of life)

- Eat plenty of fresh fruits and vegetables and other healthy food.

- Tend to your spiritual side: pray, meditate, whatever gets you back in harmony with God. Forgive any outstanding grudges.

- Stop tolerating things in your life that you don't really want. You don't have to do anything, you know.

- Say 'no' when you mean to.

- Pamper yourself each day, but at least once a week. You deserve it.

- Do something good for someone today (it's good for your soul, so you're doing it for yourself.) It could just be a smile or a good word that you say to someone.

- Take time to rest each day. You need to 'recharge' regularly.

- Delegate tasks that others can do.

- Read a good book each week. Feed your mind with useful stuff.

There are lots of other ways to help you become 'selfish' and they all serve to improve the quality of your life and inter-personal relationships. They all make you better able to serve others in ways that greatly benefit them and leave you feeling fulfilled.

Most of the tips above cost you nothing, yet they have long-lasting benefits.

A bonus tip is this: know when to seek help. Know when you need to talk to someone, to talk through things with someone. Don't keep things bottled up inside. Share your burdens either with a close friend, a family member, or a professional counsellor or coach. But never, never, never carry all your problems on your own.

Neglect yourself and you suffer for it. Why would you want to do that? You deserve to be healthy, wealthy and happy. Nobody can be those things for you, so take control of your life now.

Be selfish! (but in a good way :))

EXERCISE

GAP and write down the answers to the following:

- In what way(s) have you been neglecting yourself?

- How have you felt about yourself as a result of this?

- In what way(s) can you begin to be 'selfish'?

- In what ways do you think it would benefit you to 'love yourself' first, in the way we've described in today's chapter?

- What will you do today for yourself?

- Make a list of things you will do, and how regularly you will do them, to take care of yourself and make sure you are in good working order - physically, spiritually, emotionally.

NOTES

"You must love and care for yourself, because that's when the best comes out."
Tina Turner

DAY 24
LOVE THY NEIGHBOUR

"No man can sincerely try to help another without helping himself."
Ralph Waldo Emerson

Yesterday you read about the importance of 'loving thyself'. This makes you better able to 'love thy neighbour', so to speak. And 'who is my neighbour?' you might ask. The answer today is the same as it was over 2000 years ago when Jesus was asked the same question. Your neighbour is anyone you come across in the course of your day.

We live in a world that is populated by other human beings. We do not exist in isolation. It is therefore vital to relate with others in a way that is mutually beneficial.

The title of this article implies what is meant in the 'Golden Rule' - **'Do unto others as you would have them do unto you'**.

You would do well to make this your 'relationship mantra'. The nice thing about treating others the way we would like to be treated is that (based on the law of cause and effect), it sets good causes in motion in your life. As a result, you attract good effects to yourself whether you intend to or not.

How would you like to be treated?
Do you like to be listened to, to be understood?
Then seek to listen and understand the other person first.

Do you like to be manipulated into doing something?
If not then do not try to manipulate others into doing what you want. Check your motives before you say or do anything.

Do you like to receive compliments?
Then give compliments.

Do you like to be treated with respect?
Then treat others likewise.

Would you like to be forgiven your faults?
Then be forgiving of others' faults.

Would you like to be accepted for who you are?
Then accept others for who they are and don't try to change anybody.

Do you want to have lots of friends?
Then be friendly.

I'm sure you get the idea. If everyone practised loving each other, there will be many more happy relationships in our families, society and world. The love in question here is not some sappy, fantasy, emotional rush. I'm talking about practical love which is expressed in outward acts of kindness, goodness and all you want for yourself. Unconditional love, as opposed to the 'I'll love you if you do this that or the other'. This is the stuff that quality lives are made of.

As Erich Fromm said **"Love is the only sane and satisfactory answer to the problem of human existence."**

In any of your relationships (yes, even with the boss or colleague you 'just can't stand'), think in terms of what you can do for the other person. What can you do to make the other person's life better?

Are you in a long term relationship right now? Do you think you'd have fewer fights if you (no, let's not concern ourselves with your partner at the moment; our focus is on YOU, the only person you have the power to change…) always thought in terms of what you can give to the relationship, how you can make your partner's life better? Do you think that mindset would enrich the love between two of you and strengthen your bond?

> *"You will find as you look back upon your life that the moments when you have really lived are the moments when you have done things in the spirit of love."*
> *Henry Drummond*

Why not try it and see for yourself? It's a choice you can make. It may not be easy at first (because it goes against your natural instinct which is to hurt someone back if they hurt you) but with practice it will become second nature to you and you will have risen to a higher level of existence, a level where there is nothing but peace, joy and rest in abundance.

Are you a parent? Have you got parents? Siblings? Other relatives? Same thing applies. Especially to family. Often we take those closest to us for granted. This ought not to be the case.

The Universe is structured in such a way that you get back what you put out. If you consistently send out thoughts, words and actions of love, kindness and consideration, that is what will come back to you.

When you relate to people this way, do it with genuine concern and not with the intention of having them pay you back. Don't worry about whether or not they treat you the same way. The way things work, you WILL always be rewarded for doing the right thing, and not necessarily by the recipient of your good works either. So you can 'love your neighbour' in a detached way – not expecting anything back from them, but rather because it feels good, and is right to treat people that way.

Can you see how this sort of behaviour would enhance your life? Can you begin to imagine the level of joy and peace you would experience?

A perhaps unexpected benefit also, is that you will feel a degree of freedom you never imagined possible. This is because, when you treat others well without expecting anything back from them, you release them from owing you anything. As you release others from paying you back, so you experience release within yourself as well. It's a feeling best experienced, rather than just described.

You see, it is important for you to enjoy your stay here on earth, regardless of your pursuits and ambitions. It is important for you to have fun and be happy even as you chase your goals and dreams.

Treating people the way you'd like to be treated is a sure-fire way for you to generate true joy and peace in your life.

Benefits of that state of mind are too numerous to go into here, but realise that this sort of attitude to other people is a far more superior way of living than descending to destructive attitudes such as malice, lack of forgiveness, unresolved anger, fear, suspicion, expectation of reward or acknowledgement from others and the rest. It's just not worth it to indulge in such negative attitudes.

So love yourself: treat yourself with respect, dignity and total acceptance of who you are.

Then go out and treat everyone you come across the exact same way.

As Wayne Dyer has said, "Give love and unconditional acceptance to those you encounter and notice what happens".

EXERCISE

- What can you do from today, which you wouldn't normally do, to show love to those around you? (Family, friends, strangers, colleagues at work, church members, etc)

- GAP and write down as many ideas as you can think of and apply your ideas any time the opportunity arises.

- Write in your journal how you feel when you do so.

NOTES

"To love another person is to see the face of God."
Les Miserables

DAY 25
HOW TO OVERCOME INDECISION

*"Whatever you can do, or dream you can, begin it.
Boldness has Genius, Power and Magic in it.
Begin it now."*
Goethe

You know the feeling; we've all been there. You need to do something, but you don't know what. You are undecided about which course of action to take. It could be to do with work, your health, a relationship or any other area of life.

Consider Lorraine's situation and see if it sounds familiar. (Name changed to protect the individual concerned.)

Lorraine is a bright young woman who is stuck in a dead-end job (so she thinks), yet she is not keen to leave it. She knows she should find something else, but she doesn't know what that something else is. She has all sorts of reasons why she shouldn't take a step away from where she is, and into where she wants to be. 'I'm afraid of the unknown'; 'What if I don't like it there'; 'I don't really know what I want anyway'; 'I'll probably get another dead-end job'.

And so she remains stuck. Miserable. Sitting on the fence. Undecided. Inactive. Passive.

What is happening is actually a form of procrastination. Indecision and procrastination go hand in hand. They work together to stop you from moving ahead in your life. They keep you stuck in the same unfavourable situation you want to get out of. They keep you 'sitting on the fence.'

What situation are you tolerating in your life right now? What are you undecided about, and as a result have not made any positive progress?

Whatever it is, you need to stop sitting on the fence of indecision! The only thing you get from sitting on the fence is a sore bottom.

If you want your unfavourable circumstances to change, you've got to decide to ACT NOW. Your circumstances won't change unless you take steps to change them. Staying put won't do you any good (I guess you've figured that out by now).

As Aneurin Bevan puts it, **"We know what happens to people who stay in the middle of the road. They get run over"**

EXERCISE

How To Get Out Of The Rut

- GAP and write down what it's costing you to stay where you are now. What are you missing out on by remaining in that unfavourable job, for instance? Knowing this will make you realise how harmful it is for you to remain there. For example, you could be missing better job opportunities simply because you're not looking for them.

- Write down what you (believe you) stand to gain by staying there. What payoffs do you get? Knowing this will help you decide the benefits to look for in your new circumstance.

- Think of the big picture: where do you want to be 10 years from now? How about five years from now? Define a goal or vision for your life and write it down. Keep this goal in mind at all times.

- Brainstorm (alone or with a trusted friend) and write a list of all the options available to you which could help you reach that goal.

- For each option you've come up with:

    a. Think of the possible outcome for you if you took that path.
    b. Make lists of the pros and cons of each option.

    c. Write out the steps you need to take from where you are now to where you could be for each option.

- Now look at your final list (the one with all the info from point 5 above). Which option appeals the most to you? BEGIN NOW to take the steps you outlined above towards it. If you don't know which one appeals to you, then simply pick any one of them and begin to take steps towards it. If eventually you're not happy with where things are going, change your plans. Just don't get stuck again.

The point of this exercise is to get you off that fence and to get you to take positive steps away from your rut and into a different (and possibly better) situation.

Any action beats inaction.

So whatever you've decided to do, get off that fence and DO IT NOW!!

NOTES

"Indecision is the seedling of fear"
Napoleon Hill

DAY 26
3 STEPS TO FREEDOM

"Freedom is what you do with what's been done to you."
Jean-Paul Sartre

Have you ever noticed that it takes the same amount of time and energy to expect bad things to happen as it does to expect good things to happen?

Actually, in a lot of cases it takes more time and energy to think of negative things. So then why do many people choose to 'expect the worst'?

The reason I hear most often is that 'I'm being realistic here'. What makes you think that expecting negative outcomes to events is 'being realistic'? It's a way of disguising fear, you know. Fear that things won't turn out the way you'd really like them to. People who think that way believe they're protecting themselves from hurt. Yet what's really happening is that they're hurting their chances of getting what they do want.

I like this acronym of the word 'fear' - False Expectation Appearing Real. It summarises why it's such a waste of time expecting bad things to happen all the time.

> Sometimes if you dwell on these negative expectations long enough, they can become self-fulfilling prophecies. So be careful.

It's also a way of disguising fear of rejection, which is one of the most fundamental fears in man. You know, like when you apply for a job or when you want to ask someone out on a date and you think to yourself 'I probably won't get the job' or 'He'll probably say no'. I know you can think of other examples. This fear paralyses you into inaction – you don't bother attempting to apply for the job or ask for the date for fear you'll not get what you seek.

Yet when you don't ask for something you're 100% guaranteed not to get it...

You need to realise that thoughts are things and they do have the power to attract the very things you think of. I won't go into detail of how that happens in this chapter, but you may want to read 'The Science of Getting Rich', 'As A Man Thinketh' by James Allen and 'Think and Grow Rich' by Napoleon Hill, to give you a clearer understanding of this concept. Also 'The Power of Your Subconscious Mind' by Joseph Murphy and anything by Neville Goddard. These books are freely available online.

Your thoughts **are** things, and if the things you think about eventually come to pass in your life - which they do - doesn't it make sense to (make yourself) think about good things?

The question then arises, 'But how do I deal with disappointments? If I only expect good things to happen, how should I cope when things don't turn out as I expect?'

The answer to this lies in the following three steps (I call them the **'Three Steps To Freedom'** or simply 'The Three Steps'):

- **Expect the best** - the first step before you attempt any activity or conversation. Expect a positive, desirable outcome. Expect the best possible outcome from your efforts. If you don't, you won't be motivated to give it your best shot.

- **Be detached from the outcome** - even as you expect a good outcome, acknowledge that it could turn out either way and stay detached from the outcome. This detachment is a state of mind, an attitude you choose to adopt. The more attached you are to the outcome, the more pain you'll experience if things don't turn out the way you want. In other words, let go of the outcome. Tell yourself 'I release myself from the outcome of this task'.

- **Have faith** - believe that the outcome is for your ultimate good. If you get a different result from what you expect, believe that it's for the best. Think about it: every disappointment really is a blessing in disguise. Therefore it's all good. It's all for the best, no matter how things turn out. This faith powerfully helps you stay detached from the outcome.

God is for you, not against you. He wants only good things for you. So train yourself to live in the faith that whatever happens to you is for your ultimate good.

The verse in Romans says that **"All things work together for good to them that love God, to them who are called according to His purpose"**. When your intended outcome is a good one, rest assured that everything that happens to you on your way there is for your good, even when you don't see the immediate good in it.

The steps mentioned above are easier said than done, but it is worth every effort to practise them until they become second nature to you.

You will experience such a sense of freedom and release from pressure that you never thought was possible. This in turn puts you in the optimal state of mind to undertake any task or project you are faced with.

Besides, it's more fun to expect good things than not, isn't it?

EXERCISE

THE THREE STEPS IN ACTION
How To Apply Them

Briefly, the Three Steps are:

- Positive expectation
- Detachment from the outcome
- Faith

Here's how it works.

Positive expectation

This is easy. In any situation you're facing (and this includes personal relationships - it works beautifully here), decide the outcome you want. Then write it down in form of an expectation eg 'I expect George to be affectionate with me' or ' I expect to get this promotion'.

Next, take the appropriate action that should lead to the outcome you expect (be kind and affectionate with George; be excellent at your job).

Detachment from the outcome

This is a bit tough, so you need to decide beforehand to let go of the outcome. Acknowledge that the outcome could be positive or negative. Choose to be okay with it, whatever it is. This decision or choice is one that you make deliberately, consciously, so you're prepared for any outcome. Cultivate an attitude of 'it's all good' or 'it's for the best', regardless of the outcome. This means that you don't give up on George if he doesn't immediately respond likewise. You continue to treat him the right way, with positive expectation, but release him from the need to treat you back the right way. Release yourself also from the need to have him validate you or make you feel good about yourself. Same applies to your job. Do the best possible job you can do, not to impress your boss, but because you now operate on a higher level and you have high expectations for yourself which don't necessarily depend on your boss.

Faith

Truly believe that 'it's all good'. Using the example above, if George responds negatively, remind yourself that 'it's all good', even if you don't see the good in it at the moment. Remember, your thoughts are powerful, active things, so you want to programme yourself to have good, empowering thoughts. If George responds affectionately, tell yourself 'it's all good', too. If you don't get that promotion, remind yourself that 'it's all good'. Believe that this has happened for your ultimate good. Same thing if you do get it.

No matter how things turn out, continue to do the right thing. Keep on taking appropriate action, being flexible enough to change any action that's not leading to your intended goal.

Think of as many scenarios in your life that you can apply this principle to. It is very powerful, as people who've tried it can testify.

One major benefit of the Three Steps principle is that it helps you overcome your fears. You don't take rejection personally anymore, because you realise that 'it's all good'. It has happened for the best.

It also helps you overcome the paralysis caused by fear. You become bold, take risks and try things you've always wanted to try but have been too scared to do.

So incorporate these three steps into your life. Make them a habit from today.

NOTES

"Believe and act as though it is impossible to fail"
Charles Kettering

DAY 27

HOW TO MAKE THE MOST OF YOUR TIME

"Teach us to number our days that we may spend them wisely"
Moses

Fran (name changed) is a very talented young woman. She works as a computer network engineer, has written a novel and several short stories, loves to draw (especially comics), and has so many other things she'd like to do NOW.

Obviously, with only 24 hours in each day, during which time she has to eat and sleep, there's apparently not enough time for her to do everything she wants to do.

So what should she do? What would you do if you were in her shoes?

The phrase 'time management' comes to mind. When you think about it seriously though, it's a misnomer. You can't manage time. You can't do anything to time. **The only thing you can manage is you.**

You can manage yourself to use your time better. So I suppose the phrase 'self-management' is more appropriate.

In his book 'The Seven Habits of Highly Effective People', Steven Covey talks about four quadrants that describe our activities. His point is that our activities are either urgent (requiring immediate attention) and/or important (contributing to your mission, values and high-priority goals).

Quadrant I activities are those that are urgent and important.
Examples are deadline-driven projects. Like my weekly newsletter.

Quadrant II activities are important but not urgent. Examples are regular physical exercise, building relationships.

Quadrant III activities are urgent but not important. Examples are some phone calls or meetings.

Quadrant IV activities are neither urgent nor important. Examples are television programs, 'busy' work.

Without going into detail, the thing to recognise here is that you want your activities to be mostly quadrant II activities, and less of the others.

Quadrant II activities include writing a personal mission statement, planning and preparation.

Now let's get back to Fran above, and you if you're in a similar position. What can you do NOW to help you use your time better?

The first thing you can do is to begin to keep track of it. Start taking note of what you're doing with your time. You do have a personal mission statement, right? You called it a 'New Year's Resolution' sometime at the beginning of this year.

As you note your use of time, ask yourself which of the activities taking up your time are really necessary. Which of them contribute positively to your life and bring you closer to your goals?

Do you really need to surf the net for two hours, or have that long chat with your friend at that particular time? Dan Kennedy, in his 'No B.S. Time Management' book, talks about 'Time Vampires' – things, activities or people who suck up your time unnecessarily. You really should drive a stake through them to stop them killing your time. What are the time vampires in your life right now?

Be honest about this exercise. Awareness of a current situation is usually the first step in changing or improving it. Keep track of your time **daily** for the next seven days and see how you feel by this time next week.

The next step is to develop a plan for your life, a sort of 'big picture' of where you want to be in five or 10 years from now. A form of Mission Statement, if you will.

It's important for you to know this because it gives you a sense of direction and purpose. It also helps you prioritise your activities.

Knowing and being clear about your life mission and goal, create a list of activities that contribute to it and bring you closer to it. Prioritise this list in terms of which activities are urgent and important. Another way to prioritise it is in terms of which activities are 'A'-level priority activities. These are the ones you must do first each day, followed by 'B'-level ones, and then 'C'-level ones.

Choose the system of prioritising activities that suits you and stick to it. When you look at the activities in your time tracker, for example, using the second system, beside each one, write whether that's an A, B or C activity. Or using the first system, write beside each activity whether it's a quadrant I, II, III or IV activity.

Then rearrange your activities such that you perform more quadrant II tasks, or complete all your 'A'-level priorities first.
One thing you will discover is that you really do have time for the things that matter. We all do. After all, how come, even though we're each given 24 hours every

day, some people accomplish more than others? In the same space of time?

It boils down to how you spend the time you're given. Time is a precious commodity which once gone is lost forever.

Use yours wisely then, for you will only come by this way in life once. Use your Time Tracker to guide you and help you plan how to better utilise your time. Write down all the activities you do now, and all the ones you need to do to reach your goals. Prioritise them, make time for them and begin doing them, attending to the important things before you do the less important things.

If you need help in figuring out what's important to you, go back to the chapter on Values, read through it and reassess what your true values are. Then let them guide your goals and use of your time.

EXERCISE

For today's exercise you need your Time Tracker sheet. If you haven't downloaded yours yet, visit www.totalsuccessforwomen.com and do so now. Or create one of your own. either way, get one!

For the next seven days, keep faithful track of your time – write down exactly what you're doing at any given hour.

Decide which system for prioritising you will use – the Covey Quadrants or the A, B, C system.

When you've decided your system, classify each hourly activity into one category or the other.

At the end of each day, look at your Time Tracker sheet and think of ways to improve your use of time such that you have more Quadrant II or Category A activities in your day.

Write down your ideas for improvement and implement them the next day.

Continue with this exercise for the next seven days, and beyond, until you get into the habit of performing the important activities, the ones that definitely pull you towards your goal, first.

NOTES

*"A wise person does at once, what a fool does at last.
Both do the same thing; only at different times."*
Baltasar Gracian

DAY 28
WHY YOU SHOULD WRITE THINGS DOWN

"Writing forces you to focus. It concretises your thoughts, ideas and reflections. A goal that's not written down is merely a wish – thus, there is tremendous power in putting pen to paper."
Dr Nkem (Dr Kem) Ezeilo

By now you would have noticed that I've asked you to write something each day since we started this programme together. This has been deliberate. I have also alluded to writing in your success journal, but today, as the month draws to a close, we'll make it formal.

Something happens when you write things down. Writing crystallises your thoughts. When you decide to do something, and you write a statement of your decision, it's as if the words you have written compel you to fulfil your 'contract'.

Writing engages every part of your conscious and subconscious mind in an activity and makes you pay attention to it. That is one reason why I have asked you to write things down often in this book. If you have been doing so, you know the benefits first-hand.

If you have been following this book and taking part in the daily activities, then you probably have a well thought-out goal for your life now.

If you have been ignoring the suggested activities, why is that?

The reason you come up with is a limiting belief since it is keeping you from doing something that is certain to make your life better.

Today's lesson is about what to do with your written goals. If you do not have your goals written down somewhere, please stop reading and write them down now.

Look at your main goal every day, as often as you can, but at least twice a day. This will keep you focused on it and keep your unconscious mind working on ways to make it happen.

Write down what you need to do to bring you closer to your goal:

      a)   each month
      b)   each week
      c)   each day

Look at your monthly to-do list at the beginning of each month and break down the activities into weekly ones.

Look at your weekly to-do list at the beginning of each week and break down the activities into daily ones.

Look at your daily to-do list at the start of each day and tick off each one as you do it.
At the end of each day:

- celebrate the successful completion of the items you ticked off.

- make any necessary adjustments to the next day's to-do list.

- have a nice, peaceful and restful night.

Do not just read these things but do them. Action is the only thing that will bring about results.

The Importance of Keeping a Personal Journal

A personal journal is where you record events that occur in your day. It's a bit like a diary in that sense, except that whereas a diary is where you describe events that happened in a day, a journal includes this plus much more: your journal is where you write your reflections about the events that have happened that day: your thoughts, feelings, ideas, expectations.

Many highly successful women keep a daily journal. Take a hint and start one now. What should you write in your journal?

Anything you can think of. Write down your thoughts, your dreams, ideas, observations, anything at all. Pictures, experiences, you name it. They fit in.

The practice of keeping a journal is an important part of your self-development. There are several benefits to keeping one.

Here are a few:

- Clarifies things in your mind.
- Keeps your creative juices flowing.
- Helps you discover your true self.
- Helps you stay focused on your goals.
- Makes you better at communication (an invaluable skill).
- Has a calming, soothing effect. Things don't seem so bad when you've written them down.
- Makes your life more interesting.
- Makes you more observant of the things around you.

How long should you spend on your journal each day?

As little as five or ten minutes a day may be all you need. It's up to you. Just do it.

Again, here's something that is easy and free to do, yet it pays massive dividends in your life.

Start your daily personal journal today. Set aside at least five minutes to do it. Though you may find it so much fun you do it for longer. It's all good - just do it. Do this for the next week and see how you feel at the end of it. Then continue doing it for as long as you can.

Your journal will also provide a record of your progress in life. Without this record, you will not appreciate how far you have come. Before you leave this page, get a book and start writing down the things that are occurring to you right now.

You'll come back and thank me one day for telling you this.

EXERCISE

- Your exercise for today is to get a Success Journal and begin using it consciously, deliberately.

- Be sure to write not only events or thoughts each day, but also your feelings and ideas from them. Be free and write what you choose in this powerful little tool.

- At the end of a day's journal writing, notice how 'cleansed' and refreshed you feel. Write about that in the journal too, to remind yourself of a benefit of keeping your journal.

NOTES

"Writing in a journal reminds you of your goals and of your learning in life. It offers a place where you can hold a deliberate, thoughtful conversation with yourself.
-- Robin S. Sharma"

DAY 29
HOW TO GET RESULTS THROUGH PRAYER

"Whatsoever you desire, when you pray, believe that you receive them, and you shall have them."
Jesus Christ

This chapter will show you how to use one of the most powerful tools you have available to you in your success-creating arsenal.

That tool is prayer.

No, this has nothing to do with being religious. It has nothing to do with chanting endless, meaningless words. It does, however, have everything to do with empowering you to succeed in living a full and rich life - more than you ever believed possible.

The smartest way for you to succeed is to study successful people and copy what they do. Many successful people pray regularly. They may call it all sorts of things but it amounts to the same.

Take a hint.

Prayer is an activity that is central to your success in life. Every human being was created with the need and desire to pray. If you do not pray regularly, you are missing out on one of the most powerful experiences available to you.

What happens when you pray? Prayer is the way you communicate with that Higher Power that dwells within each of us. Some people call it the Infinite Intelligence. Others have another name for it. For brevity I'll call it God. The point is, when you pray, you are communicating with someone bigger and more powerful than yourself. You don't have to subscribe to any religion to know that you need to pray. You feel it instinctively.

The late Mahatma Gandhi called prayer "**...the most potent instrument of action**".

There is nothing mysterious about prayer – it should be as natural as breathing to you. Or at least as natural as talking to a parent. You don't need to be in a special place or position or dress in a certain way to pray effectively. You also don't need any props or special gear to do so.

Pray as you are, where you are. Just be yourself when you pray, for God knows you through and through. You don't need to put on a show. Simply pray with full faith that God exists and is willing to help you.

There's no need to complicate things. Keep it as simple as the preceding sentence has made it: pray with full faith that you already have what you are asking for. Refer to the quote at the head of this chapter.. That is the 'prerequisite' you need to fulfil in order for your prayers to be effective.

Millions of people all over the world can testify to the amazing things that happen as a result of prayer. I for one would never had tasted success if I had not prayed for it (as I continue to do).
It is said that Ralph Waldo Emerson once said **"No man ever prayed heartily without learning something"**.

What benefits do you get from praying?

You have so much to gain when you make prayer a part of your daily life. Below are a few benefits in it for you.

1. You never have to say 'there's nothing I can do about it'. **When you pray, you are doing something.** Even if you are asking for direction or for help to make the right decision, you are still doing something about your situation. With prayer, there's always something you can do.

2. You feel confident, knowing that someone bigger and more capable than you is working with you to make good things happen in your life. No team is complete without God in it. Once He's on your case, you're made.

3. Your faith increases – you begin to know that you **will** receive what you want or something better. Those are really the only options available for you when you pray with faith: you get what you ask for or you get something better. How cool is that?

4. You experience tremendous peace of mind, knowing that you are in safe hands.

5. You remain hopeful and motivated to work towards the answer to your prayer.

6. You can help people anywhere in the world when you pray for them. Awesome. This stuff works no matter where you are or who you are

7. You stay connected to the source of all that is good, the source of all that is powerful.

8. You utilise the most powerful mastermind alliance of all.

For your prayers to be effective, for them to get you the results you want, you have to fulfil certain criteria remembering the basic prerequisite mentioned above.

How To Pray So That You Get Results

I will illustrate the criteria with my experience in medical school because that was where I first successfully applied it consciously. Also, school is something a lot of people can relate to. These principles still work for me today in other areas, and I am convinced they will work for you too.

1. **Pray with a clear idea of the outcome you want**
   Be specific about what you are praying for. You want more money? State exactly how much you want. You want a job? Specify the exact position you are after. You want to lose

weight? Find a life partner? Be specific in what you are asking for. Score top grades in school? Define what you want.

When I first learned about the Universal Principles back in medical school, my specific desire was to be the best student in my class, to get top scores in all my subjects. That was exactly what happened in the end. But I had to fulfil the following criteria to make it happen.

The same applies to you. The beauty of these principles is that they work for anybody, same as God's sun shines on all.

2. **Pray with faith**
Believe that you will get what you are asking for **or something better.** Either way, you come out a winner. Remember that 'no' is an answer to prayer just as much as 'yes' is. When you pray, be absolutely certain that you will end up with the   perfect answer for you. Believe that God loves you and wants you to succeed and prosper. Believe also that God is infinitely wiser than you are, and knows what is best for you. So pray, believing that you will receive the answer that is best for you. REmember, if you believe you receive what you ask for then you shall have it.

When I prayed to excel in school, I believed that I was going to do it. I believed that so long as God was helping me, I had no option but to excel. I kept up my faith by reading the Bible (the only 'motivational' and 'inspirational' book I had then) and affirming the faith-building promises in it that   applied to me (such as 'you shall be the head and not the tail; you shall be the first and not the last' and 'if you believe that the things you say shall come to pass, you shall speak....and it will be done for you'. Powerful stuff.)

Soaking up such inspired words and affirming them while I met the criteria on this list, guaranteed my success back then and now.

3. **Behave with integrity towards everyone you meet**
   Your life has to be one that is full of good seeds and good causes set in motion. Be honest in all your dealings. Treat everyone exactly the way you would like them to treat you. Love thy neighbour. That way, when you pray, your conscience is clear. A clear conscience helps you grow and maintain your faith and self-esteem.

Back in medical school, I was always open for opportunities to help others do well in their studies too. I genuinely wanted for them what I wanted for myself, and did what I could to help them get it. Whether they did or not depended on the individuals, of course, but this attitude gave me a feeling of satisfaction and fulfilment as I pursued my goals.

4. **Speak wisely**
Your words must match your vision and your faith. In other words, if you are praying for a pay rise, for example, and you have stated the exact sum you want to receive, do not go about saying things that negate what you are praying for. Do not say things like 'I bet I won't get that rise – they passed me over last year after all'. Rather, speak words that affirm your belief and vision. Then do things that bring you closer to your vision (ie. take appropriate action).

Never speak of your vision except to confirm that it is going to happen. Your words and actions must line up with your vision and your faith, otherwise they will cancel the effect of your prayers.

Any time anyone asked me how my studies were going or how I felt about the oncoming finals, I answered in the positive. I told them I felt good about the finals, that I was going to excel in them, with God's help. The way I said it made it clear that I was not bragging, rather that I was relying on more than just my own efforts to succeed. When you have God behind you, you can literally speak things into being. It is amazing.

5. **Take Appropriate Action**
Your actions must match your vision, faith and words. There is power in that sort of congruence. Do not just pray and then sit around waiting for the answer to come. God rewards action. He will not permit you to be lazy and irresponsible if you want to prosper. He rewards appropriate action so that you become motivated to keep it up.

Remember, action brings about results. When you back your actions with prayer, you have the added advantage of gaining access to supernatural (divine) help for your tasks. You also benefit from so-called 'divine favour' – people around you feel inclined to help you out and do good things for you, often without knowing why. This phenomenon is almost eerie – takes a while to get used to it but it's one of the best feelings you could experience.

I created a study plan in school and stuck to it. During lectures, I asked questions to clarify things in my head, no matter how silly the questions sounded. Staff and students became very helpful and supportive towards me. It was as if they were going out of their way to help me reach my goals. The more I studied, the more I understood what I read. This became easier with time and it was fun too.

6. **Practice daily gratitude**
Satchel Paige, the American baseball player, said in 1974, 'Don't pray when it rains if you don't pray when the sun shines'!

Since there is a whole chapter devoted to the topic of gratitude, I will not go into more details here. Suffice it to say that an attitude of gratitude keeps you in a harmonious relationship with God, the one you pray to. Think about it: if you are a parent and your child always expresses appreciation for all you do, how would you feel if that child asks you for something? You would be inclined to do it for them, wouldn't you? Why? Because of the relationship they have maintained with you. Same thing applies here.

When you pray, be thankful for the response you are going to get, knowing that it'll be the best response for you. According to Wallace Wattles, author of the timeless classic 'The Science of Getting Rich', expressing gratitude for something that is yet to happen is the purest expression of faith.

In medical school, this was easy. As I applied the above strategies, evidence of my impending success was showing up all around me so it was easy for me to maintain gratitude. Talk about a positive success cycle.

This stuff works.

7. **Pray without ceasing**
This means you should keep your vision, your mental movie of the outcome you desire, at the forefront of your thoughts at all times. Wallace Wattles says you should spend your leisure time thinking about what you want. This is a very important step for you to follow. Don't get impatient when you don't see the results you want. Persist in prayer and action. In due time, you will succeed.

I played the 'movie' of myself going to the exam score board and seeing my top scores over and over in my head until the day it happened just like in my 'movie'. Hey what better thoughts to entertain than thoughts of me excelling, right?

8. **Meditate**
Spend time alone, in silence. During this time, think about what you want. Think about inspirational words that build your faith and motivation. While you meditate, you are likely

to receive answers to questions you have been pondering or get ideas about how to solve your problems. It is important that you take time out daily, even as little as 15 minutes per day, to just sit in silence and meditate. I got my killer study plan while meditating. It came as a thought that occurred to me as to how I should go about preparing for my multiple tasks. When the thought came, I knew it would work. And, boy, did it work. I could not have come up with such a plan on my own.

I encourage you, nay I challenge you, to pray from today, starting now. You've got absolutely nothing to lose and everything to gain when you do.

If you are serious about achieving success this year, put yourself at a huge advantage by plugging into The Source of All Success. It costs you nothing but the rewards are amazing.

Your choice.

EXERCISE

- Check your life right now.

- What is the basic prerequisite you need to have before you pray effectively?

- What are the criteria you must incorporate in your life to energise and give life to your prayers, to make them work?

- Are any of those criteria missing? If so, begin today to incorporate them into your daily programme. Be open-minded enough to give this an honest shot. I guarantee you that the results will get you hooked on prayer for good.

- Want to experience massive success in your life? Pray effectively. Don't just take my word for it.

- Do it and see.

NOTES

"Pray as though everything depended on God; Work as though everything depended on you"

St Augustine

DAY 30
YES, YOU CAN!

"If you believe you can, you probably can. If you believe you won't, you most assuredly won't. Belief is the ignition switch that gets you off the launching pad."
Denis Waitley

Congratulations! You've followed through and are here on the last day of the month. You've learnt certain blueprints for success in your life. You may still be wondering if you can apply them successfully to your life. After all, you may have tried similar techniques in the past without success.

Your inner gremlin is probably hard at work right now, trying to snuff out any motivation or inspiration you've got from this book so far. As you read today's lesson, I want you to know two things:

1. Your past does not equal your future. The fact that you have not achieved the level of success you desire does not mean you never will. Decide now that this book is the one that will make the difference for you. I have made support available to help you along the way so any time you feel stuck and need a helping hand to get you going, you know how to reach me.

2. The answer to the question 'Can you make it? Can you be truly, totally successful in any area of your life you choose?' is a resounding YES, YOU CAN!! Refuse to believe or think differently, girl!

   I am so confident and passionate about helping you own this truth for yourself that I have created a forum to provide you with ongoing support in your success journey – the Total Success For Women members' only section. I am gifting you FREE membership access to the exclusive www.totalsuccessforwomen.com site for the next 90 days as a way of (a) thanking you for purchasing this book and (b) providing ongoing encouragement, support, inspiration and motivation for you as you make these blueprints a daily way of life for yourself and (c) helping you achieve Total Success in your life!

If you could change one thing in your life today, what would it be? Why don't you have some of the things you'd like to have, and why do you have some? What's the reason for the inconsistency?

Do you find yourself wondering what people think of you? Has that line of thinking ever made you doubt your abilities and your potential?

Do you ever catch yourself thinking 'I can't do that, I'm not good enough' or 'that level of success and prosperity is for them, not for poor old me', or other similar thoughts?

One thing you must realise is that your success in any venture starts with your thoughts about it. **If you think you can succeed** (in losing weight, stopping smoking, securing a high-income job, finding your ideal partner, etc, etc), **you are already on your way to getting what you want.**

Henry Ford put it this way: **'If you think you can or if you think you can't, you're probably right'.** It's up to you to make things happen in your life.

Your mind accepts whatever you feed it as reality. Your subconscious mind does not analyse the information you feed it with, pretty much like a word processor does not analyse the information you feed it with, but rather displays it on the screen ('manifests' it) just as you've typed it into the keyboard. So if you feed it with thoughts of success (eg 'I CAN lose weight healthily', 'I CAN stop smoking', 'I CAN find a high-income job, etc, etc), it will work to make it happen.

You will become alert to opportunities (and they are all around you if you'd only open your eyes and look) to move you towards your desired results.

Conversely, if you feed your mind with negative thoughts, your mind doesn't bother to find solutions to your problems. It closes up. You wouldn't recognise an opportunity to help you out if it slapped you in the face.

You know, it takes the same amount of effort to think positive thoughts as it takes to think negative thoughts. If positive thoughts help move you towards your goals while negative ones move you further away from them, it makes sense to dwell on the positive.

Note:
Positive thinking is but a step in the journey called 'success'. You need to back your thoughts with ACTION. You can think positive thoughts until your brain gets the cramps but if all you do is think and not act, you'd be wasting your time.

> The point about positive thinking though is that it puts you in the right frame of mind to take appropriate action.

Mark Twain (and later Napoleon Hill) said that **'What the human mind can conceive and believe, the human mind can achieve'.**

The problem pops up after you've conceived your potentially great idea. The little voice inside you starts saying things like 'that's a crazy idea' or 'nobody's ever done that before - who do you think you are?' Your friends and family make fun of your idea. You begin to get discouraged and to think 'maybe it wasn't such a good idea after all'.

What should you do when this happens? Take control of your thoughts, that's what. Your mind has conceived it, remember, so your mind CAN achieve it.

You just need to line up your thoughts and actions with what you want to do.

Tell all those nay-sayers (internal and external) that you will succeed in reaching your goal.

The next line of thinking after 'I can' is 'I WILL'.

Feed yourself with thoughts like that and act accordingly - and you will see your confidence, awareness and productivity soar. You will find yourself attracting those things you want into your life.

Who says you can't make it? Tell them you CAN and you WILL. Then go out there and make it happen.

EXERCISE

You have gone through this book for the past month.

- GAP and summarise on the following page the key lesson or insight you have gained on each of the preceding days.

- What challenges have you faced as you have implemented the blueprints?

- What action steps have you successfully carried out?

- The next step is to go back to Day One tomorrow and start the course all over again. The aim of this programme is to condition you such that these blueprints become embedded in your subconscious.

- How do you feel you've done in the past month?

- What will you do differently from tomorrow?

- How will you step up your game?

- Remember to go to www.totalsuccessforwomen.com and get access to your FREE success tools today, if you haven't done so already.

NOTES

"I can do all things through Christ who gives me strength"

LAST WORD

Congratulations on coming this far in the book. Even more hearty congratulations if you have been taking action as you have read it.

Persist in your 'baby steps' and celebrate every little success you encounter as you do so. Remember, a successful life is one that is filled with days of success. A successful day is one that is filled with successful acts.

You need to be of the right mindset (healthy in spirit and mind) as well as of the right physical state (healthy in body) before you can take appropriate action that leads you to success.

Use this book as a work-out. Use it as a checklist. Use it to remind yourself of what you need to do and how you need to be in order to succeed.

Your dreams are there for a reason. Your imagination is there for a reason. Use these God-given tools to design the life you want to live. Then use the tools in this book to make them real.

God made you with more potential than you know. Don't let anybody stop you from becoming all you can be.

You will succeed. I know you will. Do you?

Go forth and prosper!

Wishing you the unlimited success you deserve,

Dr Nkem (Dr Kem) Ezeilo MBBS, Dip. Performance Coaching, MRCGP

www.totalsuccessforwomen.com

APPENDIX: HOW I OVERCAME BREAST CANCER DIAGNOSIS

I share this here not to impress you but to impress UPON you the stupendous power you have within you, for what I am able to do, so are you – the same power in me resides in you too, you've only got to plug into it.

The words and exercises in this book have pointed you in the direction of how to do this, but here's a summary of my story to show you how I applied these blueprints in my situation.

In March 2015 my breathing was bad. It had been a bit difficult earlier but I brushed it aside as I was otherwise fit and well, running 10k for charity and 5k for fitness, eating right and doing the things I was teaching others to do to stay healthy.

However when in March it got so bad that I could not run as usual, I went to get it checked out and was told that there was a massive collection of fluid around my right lung which had thus collapsed.

Turned out the fluid collection was a complication of what was diagnosed as advanced metastatic breast cancer, said to have spread from the left breast to the lungs, liver, bones. Also said to be aggressive and rapidly progressing.

None of these words fazed me because I knew that no matter what was said about me, it's what I chose to believe about me that came to pass, meaning that if I chose to believe what they had just said about me, then their prognosis would come to pass.

So I chose to believe that death and life are in the power of my tongue, not in the power of the doctors or test results. Believing this, I started to speak life into my body. You could say that my 'goal' was to live long and healthy. Still is.

Of course I wondered how the heck I had come to be experiencing this, being a 'Health guru' and all. In fact I had been on a plant based diet when this diagnosis hit. Ongoing through my personal 10 Pillars of Health, I came to realize that the pillar that was weak, which led to this diagnosis, was my First Pillar: I had some serious unresolved emotional issues. Had been so busy helping others sort through their issues, and helping others achieve success and improve their lives, working crazy hours as a doctor for years, I literally had not had time to address certain emotionally traumatic experiences I'd gone through years earlier in my life.

When you seek (a cause) you will find one.

When you ask (a question) you will receive an answer.

The key thing I want you to understand and remember is that my belief in my body's ability to heal itself, my belief in the power of my words to keep me alive and well, my belief is what fuels my actions and words leading to my still being here today.

My belief is that I will live long enough to see my son's grandchildren.

So every day I am given, more than ever, I value and appreciate for I know that many people in similar position have believed the words of the doctors or test reports, and have died as predicted by those well meaning people.

I encourage you – own your own power.

Nobody has any power over you unless you give it to them.

No condition has any power over you unless you give it to it.

Remember the chapter on 'The Power To Choose'? That chapter is very important (as are all the others) because it reveals the one thing that makes you more powerful than you could possibly understand or imagine.

I exercise my power to choose liberally every day. Every day I wake up, I choose to be thankful . I am thankful for life and more of it. I am thankful just for the sake of being thankful. I choose to live. Yes, life is a choice I make every day – you've got to make conscious choices each day for your choices carry consequences that you have to deal with, so it's important to make the choices you make ones whose consequences you are proud of. I choose to be happy each day.

So yes I was given that diagnosis. I choose my words around this and I say that I was given the diagnosis. I never say 'I have cancer', for that is not my reality. My reality is that I have life and health. The diagnosis is something that was given to me. I rejected the diagnosis and its implications and my body is fast catching up to that reality that I am perfectly healthy and alive.

You see, your body does respond to your thoughts and beliefs and words. So it's important that you are careful what these are.

I encourage you by my story, to take control of your life. You are nobody's slave unless you choose to be. No matter what you've been through, no matter what you've been called, no matter what, you can overcome any challenge life brings your way. You really are that special, that amazing, that awesome, that powerful.

The entire creative force that birthed the universe, is WITHIN you.
- The Kingdom of heaven is in you

- He that is in you is greater than whatever is outside you
- The power in you is able to do exceedingly above, and beyond all you could ever possibly ask or think...
- You can do ALL things through the Christ in you.

Need I go on? Do you now begin to realize just how powerful you are?

This power goes by various names: God, Subconscious Mind, Imagination, Christ, Universe, Higher Power – of a truth it doesn't give a hoot what you call it. All that matters is that you recognize and use it to create the life you desire.

I've not even fully grasped this power within me, but the little I know and have acted on, is working wonders for me. Can you imagine unleashing the full power? People call it 'miracle', but that's really the way we were designed to operate.

Own your power. It's your birthright. Use it to life life to the fullest as you were created to do.

Here's to your successful, fulfilling, joyful future...

ABOUT THE AUTHOR

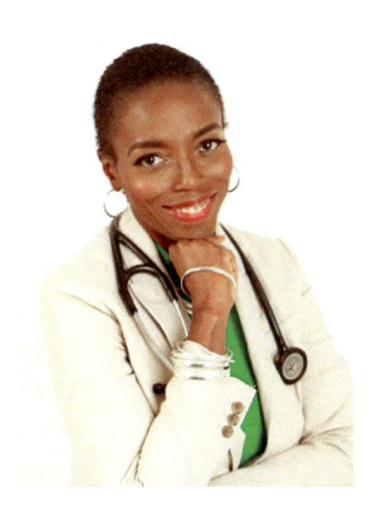

Dr Nkem Ezeilo, fondly called "Dr Kem", is a woman who is passionate about "making women's lives better". Right from when she was very young, she wanted to help people stop suffering and lead happy and fulfilling lives. It was no surprise then that she chose medicine as a career. This gave her ample opportunity to work personally with people in need, and watch them recover under her care.

It was in medical school that Dr Kem learnt to apply the Universal Principles of Success she teaches today. This is a woman who knows first hand what it means to succeed. After a string of mediocre grades in medical school, she stumbled upon the 'secret' to success and excellence in academics. This made a huge difference in her outlook and performance in academics as well as life from then onwards.

She graduated from medical school with distinctions in every subject, winning several awards including 'Best Overall Medical Student 1997'.

Having decided to start a family, she put her promising medical career on hold to raise her son-her most rewarding role yet. While at home, and wanting to fulfil her lifelong desire to help others improve, Dr Kem trained as a Life Coach and began to consult from home, helping clients to accomplish goals they had not been able to achieve before.

Using the Universal Principles of Success, Dr Kem built her coaching practice into an international organisation, with clients phoning in from various continents.

After being away from medicine for a total of 7 years, Dr Kem returned to medical practice and successfully completed a post graduate specialty training program in General Practice, becoming a member of the prestigious Royal College of General Practitioners, UK.

Dr Kem uses the success principles shared in this book to overcome any challenges life brings her way. She has used them to overcome breast cancer twice, the second time being the worst possible diagnosis where she was not expected to live beyond 3 months. However by engaging the incredible power of the mind, Dr Kem has overcome this and is now committed to showing others how they too can overcome life's obstacles no matter how serious.

Today, she works tirelessly to share these principles with women, teaching them how to fulfil their true potential and accomplish tasks they initially thought were beyond them.

Contact Dr Kem today with any feedback or comments by sending a message on the 'Contact Us' page at www.totalsuccessforwomen.com

Miscellaneous

- Dr Kem is available (depending on her schedule) to speak to, coach and train individuals and organizations on the thinking skills needed to succeed in today's world. To find out more, and to book Dr Kem to speak at your event, please fill in the contact form over at www.totalsuccessforwomen.com

- Subscribe to the FREE electronic newsletter 'Weekly Success Tips for Women' by visiting www.totalsuccessforwomen.com